Textbook of PATHOLOGY AND GENETICS for BSc Nursing Students

Chaitra K MBBS DCP
Consultant Pathologist and Laboratory Head
SRL Diagnostics Ltd. Fortis Hospital, Nagarbhavi
Bengaluru, Karnataka, India

Suma K MBBS DCP
Consultant Pathologist
Bengaluru, Karnataka, India

Forewords
Leena Chatterjee
Nagarajappa AH

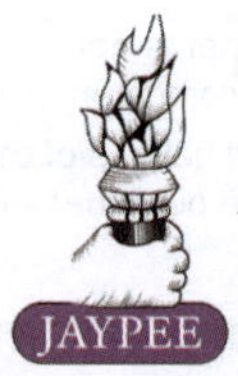

JAYPEE BROTHERS MEDICAL PUBLISHERS
The Health Sciences Publisher
New Delhi | London

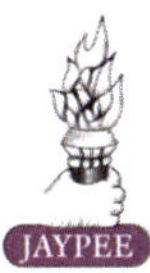

Jaypee Brothers Medical Publishers (P) Ltd

Headquarters
EMCA House
23/23-B, Ansari Road, Daryaganj
New Delhi 110 002, India
Landline: +91-11-23272143, +91-11-23272703
+91-11-23282021, +91-11-23245672
E-mail: jaypee@jaypeebrothers.com

Corporate Office
Jaypee Brothers Medical Publishers (P) Ltd.
4838/24, Ansari Road, Daryaganj
New Delhi 110 002, India
Phone: +91-11-43574357
Fax: +91-11-43574314
E-mail: jaypee@jaypeebrothers.com

Overseas Office
JP Medical Ltd.
83, Victoria Street, London
SW1H 0HW (UK)
Phone: +44-20 3170 8910
Fax: +44(0)20 3008 6180
E-mail: info@jpmedpub.com

Website: www.jaypeebrothers.com
Website: www.jaypeedigital.com

Inquiries for bulk sales may be solicited at: jaypee@jaypeebrothers.com

Textbook of Pathology and Genetics for BSc Nursing Students

First Edition: 2016
Reprint : **2024**
ISBN: 978-93-5152-817-3

Printed in India at Rajkamal Electric Press, Kundli, Haryana-131 028

Dedicated to

My husband, Mr Harsha,
my daughter Inchara, my parents and
my sister for their everlasting encouragement,
love and support

—Chaitra K

My greatest inspiration Abhinav,
my husband Dr (Col) Madhu PV, my son Pranav,
my parents and brother whose encouragement and
unwavering support were essential to the successful preparation
and completion of this book

—Suma K

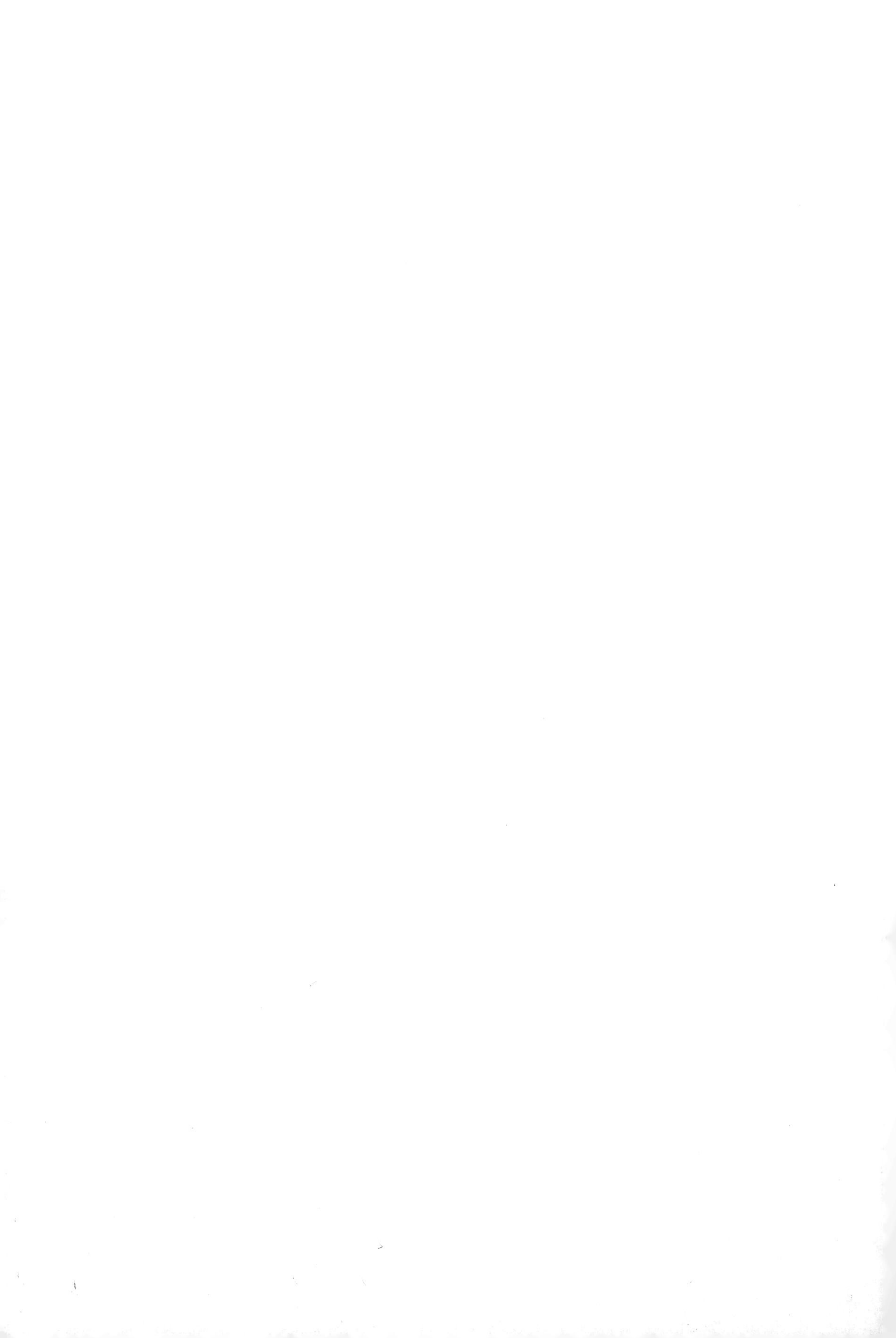

Foreword

I am delighted at being asked to write the foreword and be a part of the *Textbook of Pathology and Genetics for BSc Nursing Students*.

Dr Chaitra K and Dr Suma K are both dedicated and sincere pathologists who earlier worked at Bangalore Medical College and Research Institute, Bengaluru, Karnataka, India, and have moved on to being efficient Consultant Pathologists today. Dr Chaitra K works as a Consultant Pathologist and Laboratory Head at SRL Diagnostics Ltd., Fortis Hospital, Bengaluru, Karnataka, India. Dr Suma K is working as a freelance Consultant Pathologist. Both of them have an in-depth understanding of the basics of Pathology and great interest in academics.

The subjects Pathology and Genetics are very important parts of BSC nursing. The knowledge as to 'why' and 'how' diseases occur and how they progress is vital for every budding nurse to understand. This book presents the topics in a very comprehensive way and helps the students understand the basics of Pathology. Written in accordance with the syllabus prescribed by the Indian Nursing Council (INC), this textbook uses very simple language with pictorial representation wherever necessary. Another highlight of the book is the line diagrams which have been digitized and are very easy to understand.

I wish the authors luck and success for their future endeavors; and, I also wish this textbook, the academic reach with students that it is deserving of. I hope the students of Nursing enjoy reading this textbook.

Leena Chatterjee
Director
Fortis SRL Labs and SRL Strategic Initiatives
SRL Limited
(Global Diagnostics Network)
New Delhi, India

Foreword

I am happy to write the foreword for the *Textbook of Pathology and Genetics for BSc Nursing Students* authored by two brilliant Pathologists, Dr Chaitra K and Dr Suma K. I am happy to be associated with both of them since they were tutors at Bangalore Medical College and Research Institute, Bengaluru, Karnataka, India. They are both very dedicated and multitalented. The textbook is comprehensive and covers all the chapters according to the syllabus prescribed by the Indian Nursing Council (INC). I wish Dr Chaitra and Dr Suma good luck in their future endeavors.

Nagarajappa AH
Former Professor and Head
Department of Pathology
Bangalore Medical College and Research Institute
Bengaluru, Karnataka, India

Preface

We are delighted to introduce the *Textbook of Pathology and Genetics for BSc Nursing Students*.

There was a felt need for a concise and comprehensive book on Pathology and Genetics for the reference by students. We have brought this material together in a cohesive and organized fashion. The book is in accordance with the syllabus prescribed by the Indian Nursing Council for the students.

The book contains the information needed in a simple and easily understandable language. The chapters in General Pathology are made easier by the addition of diagrammatic representations and tables. The chapters on Systemic Pathology contain many gross and microscopic pictures that make the reading more interesting. The chapters on Clinical Pathology and Genetics complete the discussion on the subject.

It is our sincere wish that you find this book informative and helpful. We ensure that this will be an excellent resource and will appeal to all the nursing students.

Chaitra K
Suma K

Acknowledgments

We are grateful to many people who have contributed in many ways towards the completion of this book.

We offer our sincere thanks to Dr Nagarajappa AH, Former Professor and Head, Department of Pathology, Bangalore Medical College and Research Institute, Bengaluru, Karnataka, India, for encouraging us in this endeavor. We are deeply indebted to him for writing the foreword for this book. We also express our heartfelt thanks to Dr Leena Chatterjee, Director, Fortis SRL Labs and SRL Strategic Initiatives, SRL Limited (Global Diagnostics Network), New Delhi, India for penning the foreword for this book.

Special thanks to M/s Jaypee Brothers Medical Publishers (P) Ltd., New Delhi, India, for believing in us, encouraging us to write the book and turning it into a reality by publishing it.

We express our gratitude to Dr (Col) Madhu PV for writing the chapter on Fluid and Electrolyte Imbalance. Our heartfelt thanks to Mr Harsha M for helping us in scanning the pictures and for the constant technical support.

We are thankful to all our colleagues, especially Dr Reshma A and Dr Priyadarshini N for their support.

Final word of gratitude to all our family members and friends who have encouraged us directly and indirectly in bringing out this book.

Contents

Section 1 Pathology

Section 2 Genetics

SECTION 1

Pathology

CHAPTER 1

Introduction

Pathology is a branch of medicine that deals with the systematic and scientific study of the disease.

The exact meaning of the word pathology is study (logos) of the suffering (pathos).

Pathology involves the structural and functional changes in the cells, tissues and organs that are diseased. The progression and outcome of a particular disease is based on the cellular and molecular changes within the cell. The knowledge of these changes assists in the clinical diagnosis and treatment.

Pathology is divided into various segments, for the purpose of study as general pathology, systemic pathology, hematology and clinical pathology.

The study of any disease process involves four different concepts, which includes:

1. Etiology
2. Pathogenesis
3. Morphologic changes
4. Functional derangements and clinical manifestations.

ETIOLOGY

Etiology means the "Cause". It deals with finding out what caused the disease? Or, why the disease has occurred? The factors which are responsible for causing the disease are called etiologic factors. In general, the etiologic agents can be divided into intrinsic/genetic and acquired.

PATHOGENESIS

From the time the cell/tissue is exposed to a particular etiologic agent, various changes occur in it to ultimately produce the disease. The occurrence of these sequences of events in the cell/tissue is called pathogenesis.

MORPHOLOGIC CHANGES

Morphologic changes refer to the structural changes which occur in the diseased cell/tissue and involve two things.

Gross

The macroscopic appearance of the diseased tissue to the naked eye are called gross examination (Fig. 1.1).

Microscopy

The changes seen in the diseased cells or tissues under the microscope is called microscopic examination (Fig. 1.2).

FUNCTIONAL DERANGEMENTS AND CLINICAL MANIFESTATIONS

Once a particular organ is diseased, its normal functioning capacity is reduced or altered. This will result in deviation from the normal, and

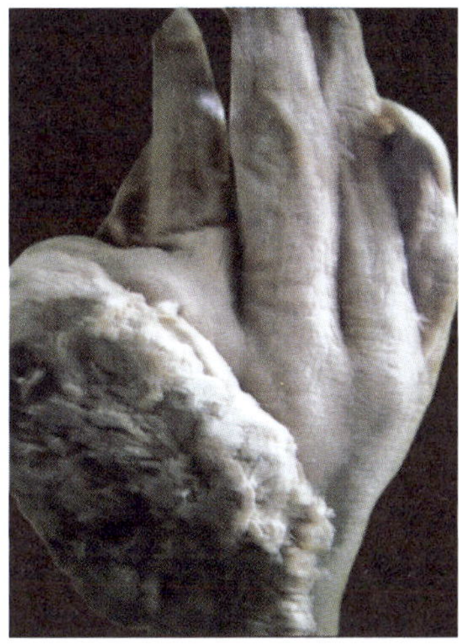

FIGURE 1.1 Gross appearance of squamous cell carcinoma as it appears to the naked eye

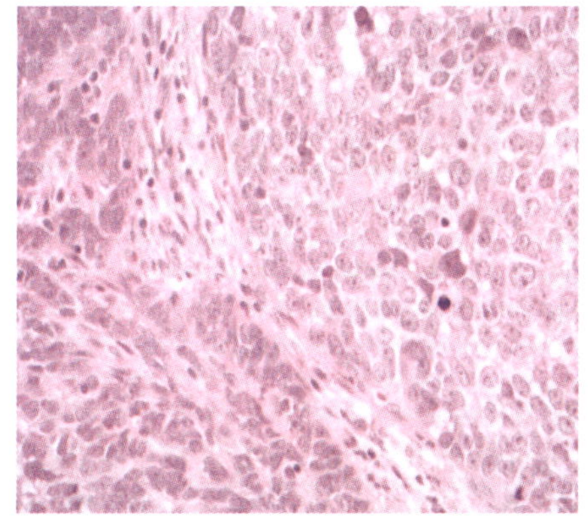

FIGURE 1.2 Microscopic appearance of squamous cell carcinoma

cause the specific signs and symptoms of that particular disease.

CELLULAR AND TISSUE CHANGES

Cellular Adaptations

The normal cell in our body works to handle the normal physiologic demands. But severe physiologic stress and sometimes pathologic stimuli, results in cellular adaptations.

Cellular adaptation can be defined as a process by which new, altered but steady structural and functional state is reached by the cell.

Hyperplasia

It is an adaptive change where there is an increase in the number of cells. It can be physiological or pathological.

Physiologic hyperplasia can be due to hormonal stimulation when there is an extra demand as in the pregnant uterus or pubertal growth of breasts in females. The other form of physiologic hyperplasia is the compensatory hyperplasia, where there is an increased growth due to loss or absence of a particular organ. The example is the compensatory hyperplasia seen in the remaining kidney after one kidney has been removed.

Pathologic hyperplasia is due to unnecessary excessive hormonal stimulation on the target organ. An example for this is endometrial hyperplasia due to excessive estrogen stimulation, which leads to abnormal menstrual bleeding. This hyperplasia though abnormal, will revert back to normal once the hormonal stimulation is stopped. This property of reversibility is the one which distinguishes pathologic hyperplasia from cancer.

Hypertrophy

Hypertrophy is an adaptive response that involves increase in the size of the cell, but the number remains constant. The increase in the size of the cell is due to an increase in the synthesis of cellular organelles. As in hyperplasia, it can also be either physiological or pathological.

Physiologic hypertrophy is due to increased workload. The classical example is that of hypertrophied biceps and triceps muscles in body builders, uterus in pregnancy also hypertrophies to a great extent.

Pathologic hypertrophy is seen in heart muscles of inpatients suffering from hypertension or stenotic heart valves.

Atrophy

Atrophy is an adaptive response in which there is a decrease in the size and function of the cells. It causes cell shrinkage, due to loss of cell substance.

Physiologic atrophy is seen in early age, during embryogenesis in the fetus, where there is atrophy of the notochord and thyroglossal duct. The reduction in the size of uterus shortly after childbirth is another example of physiologic atrophy.

Pathologic atrophy can be due to a variety of causes. It can be due to reduced workload (disuse atrophy), due to loss of innervation (denervation atrophy), due to loss of blood supply or inadequate nutrition, due to aging (senile atrophy) or due to loss of hormonal stimulation.

Metaplasia

Metaplasia is a reversible change in which one adult cell type (epithelial or mesenchymal) is replaced by another adult cell type. It is an adaptive response where the body switches over to the type of cell which can withstand the stress well in adverse conditions.

Examples: Epithelial metaplasia—columnar epithelium is replaced by squamous epithelium in respiratory tract due to chronic irritation, commonly seen in smokers.

Mesenchymal metaplasia: Bone is seen in the muscle occasionally after fracture and is designated as myositis ossificans.

Dysplasia

Dysplasia means disordered growth. It usually progresses to neoplasm, if not treated. This is explained in detail in the chapter on Neoplasia (Chapter 2).

CELL INJURY

Cell injury results when the limits of adaptive responses are crossed beyond a particular point, with the inciting stress still being present. The cell injury can be reversible or irreversible (cell death) (Fig. 1.3).

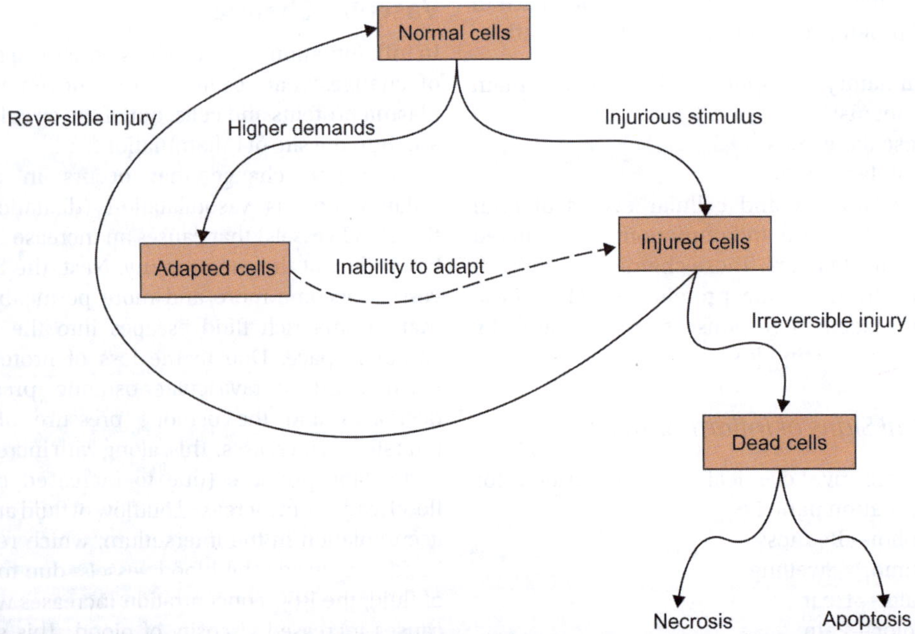

FIGURE 1.3 Cell injury

INFLAMMATION AND REPAIR

Inflammation

Definition

"Inflammation is a complex reaction to injurious agents such as microbes and damaged, necrotic cells that consist of vascular responses, migration and activation of leukocytes and systemic reaction."

Stated in a simple way, " Inflammation is the response of a living tissue to an injury."

Regeneration and Repair

The inflammatory response is closely related with the process of repair. The injured tissue, during repair is replaced through replacement of the native parenchymal cells.

Depending on the duration of response of tissue to the injurious stimuli, it can be divided into:

- *Acute inflammation:* Rapid response to injurious agent (within seconds, minutes, hours or few days).
- *Chronic inflammation:* It is the inflammation of prolonged duration of weeks or months.

Inflammatory response has two main components:

1. Vascular events
2. Cellular events.

The vascular and cellular events of both acute and chronic inflammation are mediated by chemical factors. These chemical factors are derived from plasma proteins or cells. These are produced in response to or activated by inflammatory stimulus.

Clinical Signs of Inflammation

There are five classical signs described for inflammation namely:

1. Rubor—Redness
2. Tumor—Swelling
3. Calor—Heat
4. Dolor—Pain
5. Functio laesa—Loss of function.

Acute Inflammation

Acute inflammation is rapid in onset (within seconds or minutes) and lasts for a short duration of minutes, several hours and a few days.

It has three major components:

1. Increase in the flow of blood to the injured tissue.
2. Structural changes in the blood vessels that permit plasma proteins and WBCs to leave the circulation.
3. Migration and accumulation of WBCs at the site of injury and their activation to remove the offending agent.

Stimuli for Acute Inflammation

1. Infections—Bacteria, virus, parasites
2. Trauma
3. Burns, irradiation, frostbite
4. Tissue necrosis
5. Foreign bodies such as suture material, splinters, dirt, etc.
6. Immune reactions.

Vascular Changes

In inflammation, blood vessels undergo a series of changes that results in the movement of plasma proteins and cells, out of the circulation and into the site of inflammation.

The first change that occurs in acute inflammation is vasodilatation (dilatation of the blood vessels) that causes an increase in the blood flow at the site of injury. Next, the blood vessels become more and more permeable so that plasma rich fluid escapes into the extra vascular space. Due to the loss of protein in plasma, the intravascular osmotic pressure decreases and the osmotic pressure of the interstitium increases. This, along with increased hydrostatic pressure (due to increased blood flow) leads to an increased outflow of fluid and its accumulation in the interstitium, which results in edema. Inside the blood vessels, due to loss of fluid, the RBC concentration increases which causes increased viscosity of blood. This slows down the blood flow and is called stasis (Fig. 1.4).

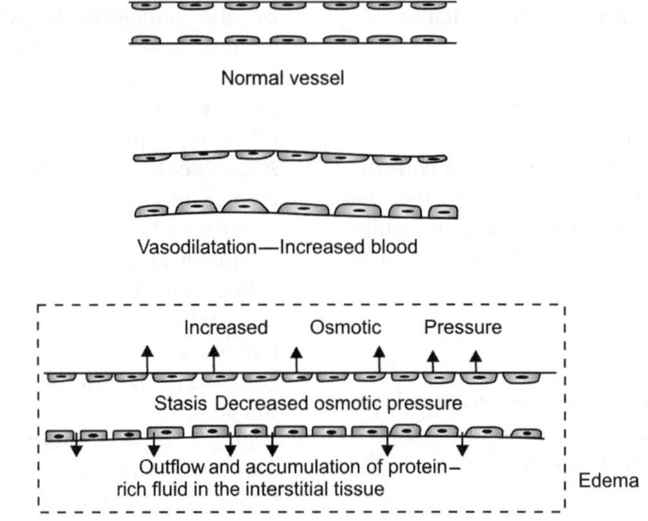

FIGURE 1.4 Diagrammatic representation of vascular changes in acute inflammation

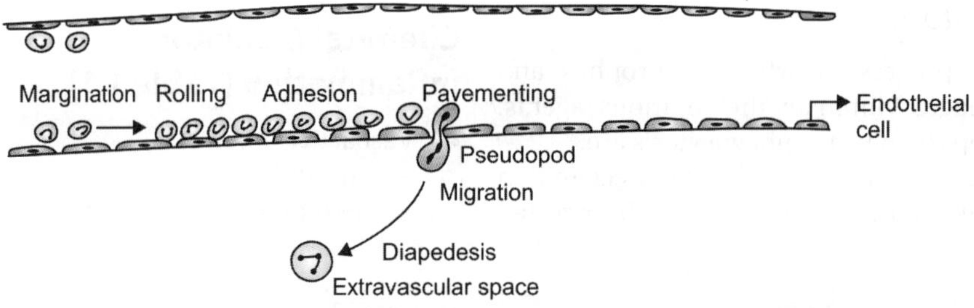

FIGURE 1.5 Diagrammatic representation of cellular events in inflammation

Cellular Changes

Inflammation results in accumulation of WBCs at the site of injury and their activation. These activated WBCs ingest the offending agents, kill the bacteria and virus and get rid of necrotic tissue and foreign substances.

Extravasation

It is the sequence of events in the journey of WBCs from the blood vessel lumen into the interstitial tissue towards the site of inflammation. It includes the following:

1. *Margination:* In inflammation, due to stasis in the blood vessel lumen, the WBCs move towards the periphery. They take a position along the endothelial surface. This process is called margination.
2. *Rolling:* Next, the WBCs slip down the endothelial cells finally coming to rest at some point where they adhere firmly. This process is called 'rolling'.
3. *Pavementing:* In time, endothelium is virtually lined by a row of WBCs and is called pavementing.
4. *Adhesion and migration:* The WBCs firmly adhere to the endothelium by means of adhesion molecules. Then, they insert pseudopods into the junction between the endothelial cells, squeeze through the endothelial junction and eventually migrate into the extravascular space (Fig. 1.5).

There are four types of adhesion molecules:

1. Selectins.
2. Integrins.
3. Immunoglobulin family of molecules.
4. Mucin-like glycoproteins.

The type of WBC migrating varies with the type of inflammation. Initially, during the first six to 24 hours, it is dominated by neutrophils. Later, monocytes take over in the next 24 to 48 hours.

Chemotaxis

It is a process by which WBCs immigrate in tissue towards the site of injury. Chemoattractant is a substance which attracts the WBCs towards the site of injury. It can be exogenous like bacterial products or endogenous like components of complement system.

Phagocytosis

It is the process by which neutrophils and macrophages eliminate the injurious agents. Three steps involved in phagocytosis are:

1. *Recognition and attachment:* Recognition and attachment of the particle to be ingested by the leukocyte by specific receptors expressed on its surface. Opsonins are specific proteins which are expressed on the particle to be ingested and it increases the efficiency of phagocytosis.
2. *Engulfment:* The WBCs extend the cytoplasm in pseudopods around the particle to be engulfed. This results in the complete enclosure of the particle and is called the phagosome. This phagosome binds with the lysosomal granule inside the leukocyte to form the phagolysosome. The contents of the granule are discharged into the phagolysosome.
3. *Killing and degradation:* Activation of the phagocyte (leukocyte) will result in ultimate killing and degradation of the offending agent. This is done by oxygen dependent and oxygen independent mechanisms (Fig. 1.6).

Chemical Mediators of Inflammation (Table 1.1)

- Vasoactive amines
  - Histamine
  - Serotonin

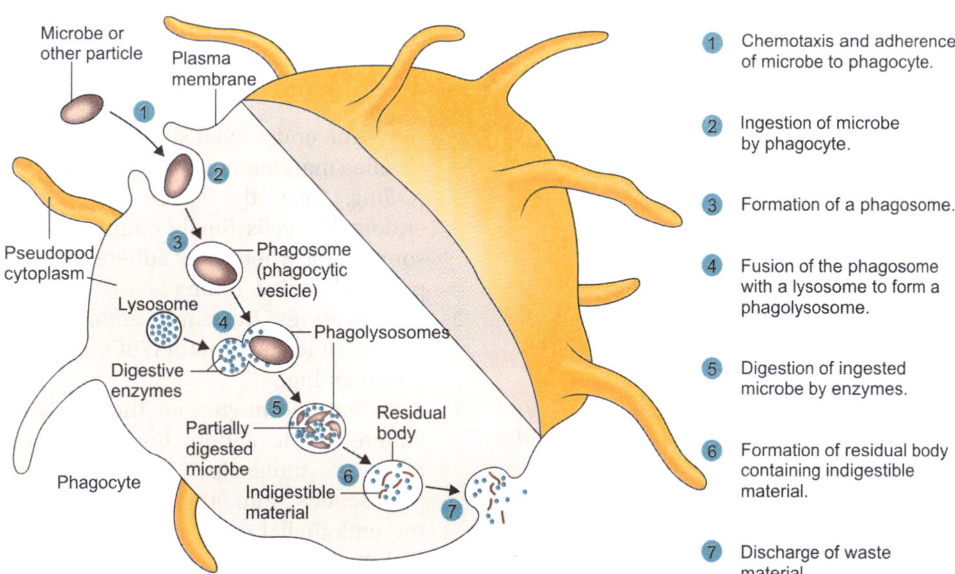

FIGURE 1.6 Diagrammatic representation of phagocytosis

TABLE 1.1 Role of mediators in different reactions of inflammation	
Vasodilatation	Prostaglandins Nitric oxide Histamine
Increased vascular permeability	Vasoactive amines C3a and C5a Bradykinin Leukotrienes C4, D4, E4
Chemotaxis, leukocyte recruitment and activation	C5a Chemokines Bacterial products
Fever	Interleukin 1 Tumor necrosis factor Prostaglandins
Pain	Prostaglandins Bradykinin
Tissue damage	Neutrophil and macrophage lysosomal enzymes

- Plasma proteins
  - Complement system
  - Kinin system
  - Clotting system
- Arachidonic acid metabolites
  - Prostaglandins
  - Leukotrienes
  - Lipoxins
- Platelet-activating factor
- Cytokines and chemokines
- Nitric oxide
- Lysosomal constituents of leukocytes
- Oxygen derived free radicals
- Neuropeptides.

Histamine

- *Source*: Mast cell, basophil, and platelet.
- Released in response to a variety of stimuli like trauma, cold, heat, immune reactions, anaphylaxis, neuropeptides and cytokines.
- Histamine causes dilatation of the arterioles and increases the permeability of venules.

Complement System

The complement system has about 20 complement components which are found in greatest concentration in plasma. They cause increased vascular permeability, chemotaxis and opsonization which help in inflammation.

Other cells involved in chronic inflammation are:
- *Lymphocytes:* These are seen in both humoral and cell-mediated immunity.
- *Eosinophils:* These are abundant in parasitic infections and IgE mediated immune reactions.
- *Mast cells:* Usually seen in response to anaphylactic reactions.

GRANULOMATOUS INFLAMMATION

Granulomatous inflammation is a distinctive pattern of chronic inflammation characterized by the formation of granulomas. A granuloma is a focus of chronic inflammation consisting of a microscopic aggregate of epithelioid cells (modified macrophages having an epithelium-like appearance) surrounded by lymphocytes and occasional plasma cells.

Epithelioid cell can be described as a modified macrophage which is elongated with pale pink granular cytoplasm with indistinct cell borders and slipper shaped oval nucleus.

Older granulomas develop a rim of fibroblasts and connective tissue. Giant cells are formed by the fusion of epithelioid cells.

Giant Cells

There are different types of giant cells:
- *Langhan's giant cell:* Multiple nuclei are arranged peripherally in a horseshoe like arrangement. Seen in tuberculosis.
- *Foreign body giant cell:* Multiple nuclei arranged haphazardly inside the cell.
- *Tumor giant cell:* Nuclei of varying sizes arranged haphazardly.
- *Osteoclastic giant cell:* Up to 100 nuclei of the same size scattered in the cytoplasm.

MORPHOLOGY

Characteristics of chronic inflammation are:

- Infiltration with mononuclear cells, which includes macrophages, lymphocytes and plasma cells.
- Tissue destruction.
- Attempts at healing by connective tissue replacement of damaged tissue, accomplished by proliferation of small blood vessels (angiogenesis) and fibrosis.

Mononuclear Cell Infiltration

Macrophage is the hallmark cell of chronic inflammation. These macrophages in tissue are called by different names like Kupffer cells in the liver, sinus histiocytes in the spleen and lymph node and alveolar macrophages in the lungs.

As discussed previously, blood monocytes are the dominant cells to migrate to the site of inflammation at 48 hours. When the monocyte reaches the tissue, it undergoes transformation into macrophages. These macrophages are activated by a variety of stimuli like cytokines, bacterial toxins and other chemical mediators. The activated macrophage has a greater ability to phagocytose and kill ingested microbe. In chronic inflammation, the accumulation of macrophage persists by different mechanisms:

- Recruitment of monocytes from circulation
- Local proliferation of macrophage
- Immobilization of macrophages

The products of activated macrophages serve to eliminate injurious agents such as microbes and to initiate the process of repair and are responsible for tissue injury caused in chronic inflammation. The enzymes produced by macrophages also have the potential to digest the extracellular matrix. Thus, tissue destruction is the hallmark of chronic inflammation.

Examples of granulomatous inflammation:

- *Immune granuloma:* It is caused by microbes. The phenotype of immune granuloma is tuberculosis. This is charac terized by classic picture of central caseous necrosis, surrounded by epithelioid cells and lymphocytes along with Langhan's giant cells.
- *Foreign body granuloma:* It is initiated by inert foreign body. Typically foreign body granuloma forms to talc or suture material.

CUTANEOUS WOUND HEALING

Cutaneous wound healing is divided into three phases:

1. Inflammation.
2. Granulation tissue formation and re-epithelialization.
3. Wound contraction, extracellular matrix deposition and remodeling (Table 1.2).

TABLE 1.2 Cutaneous wound healing

Time	*Changes seen in the wound*
Within 24 hours	Neutrophils at the margin of the incision moving towards the fibrin clot
24 to 48 hours	Spurs of epithelial cells move from wound edges along the cut margins, depositing basement membrane material. This continuous layer closes the wound
Day 3	Neutrophils are replaced by macrophages. Granulation tissue is produced
Day 5	Incision space is filled with granulation tissue. Abundant collagen bridges the incision. Epidermis matures with surface keratinization
During second week	Continued accumulation of collagen and proliferation of fibroblasts
By the end of first month	Scar made of cellular connective tissue devoid of inflammatory infiltrate Intact epidermis is present. The dermal appendages in the line of incision are permanently lost. After several months, the tensile strength in the wound area increases

Skin wounds are classically described to heal by primary or secondary intention.

Healing by Primary Intention (Wounds with Opposed Edges)

The best example is that of a clean, uninfected, surgical incision approximated by surgical sutures. Such healing is called healing by primary intention. The sequence of events in this process is described in Figure 1.7.

Healing by Second Intention (Wounds with Separated Edges)

When there is extensive loss of cells and tissue, these wounds create a large defect. Healing in such wounds involve formation of abundant granulation tissue to fill the defect. Large tissue defects generate a large fibrin clot and more necrotic debris that must be removed. So, the inflammatory reaction is more intense. Wound contraction is an important feature

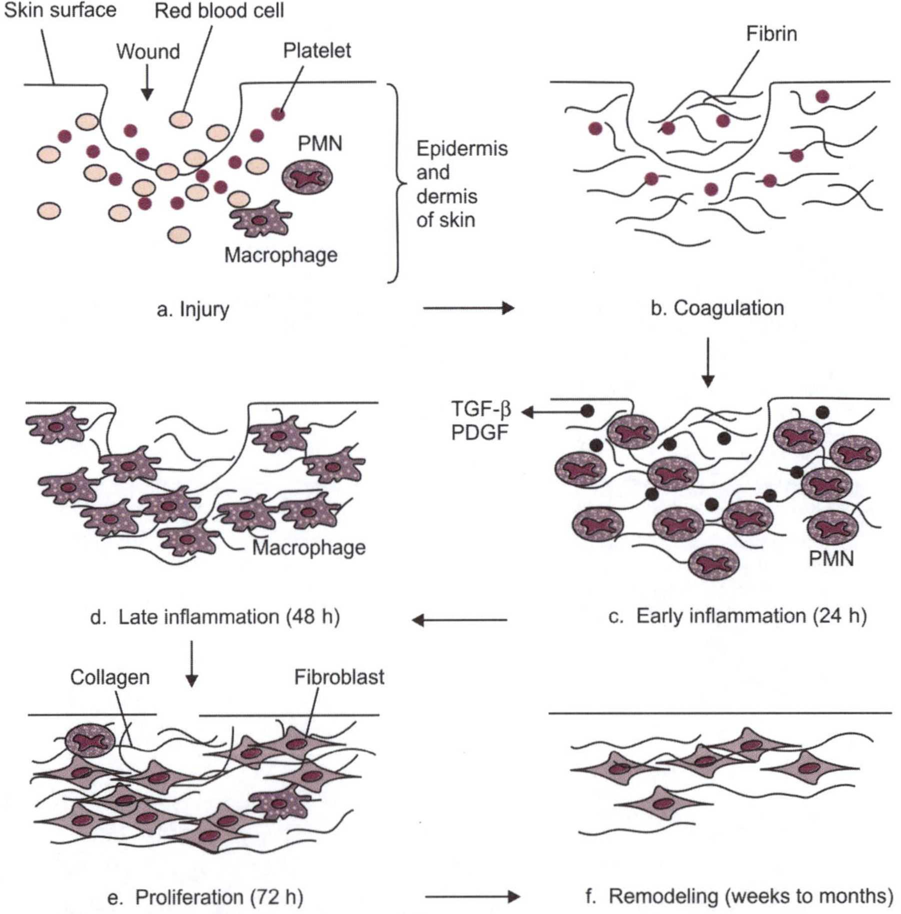

FIGURE 1.7 Diagrammatic representation of different steps in wound healing by primary intention

TABLE 1.3 Factors that retard wound healing

Local factors	*Systemic factors*
Blood supply	Age
Denervation	Anemia
Local infection	Drugs
Foreign body	Genetic disorders
Hematoma	Hormones
Mechanical stress	Diabetes
Necrotic tissue	Malignant disease
Surgical techniques	Malnutrition, obesity
Type of tissue	Systemic infection

that differentiates it from healing by primary intention. This leads to large scar formation and thinning of the epidermis.

FACTORS INFLUENCING WOUND HEALING (TABLE 1.3)

Complications of Cutaneous Wound Healing

- Deficient scar formation
- Excessive formation of granulation tissue
- Formation of contractures.

CHAPTER 2

Neoplasia

Neoplasia means "new growth". *Oncology* (In Greek, *oncos* = tumor) is the study of tumors or neoplasms. Cancer is the common term for all malignant tumors.

The eminent British oncologist Sir Rupert Willis has given the definition:

"A neoplasm is an abnormal mass of tissue, the growth of which exceeds and is uncoordinated with that of the normal tissues and persists in the same excessive manner after cessation of the stimuli which evoked the change."

All tumors have two basic components:

1. Proliferating neoplastic cells that constitute their parenchyma.
2. Supportive stroma made up of connective tissue and blood vessels.

Sometimes the parenchymal cells stimulate the formation of an abundant collagenous stroma, referred to as desmoplasia.

Benign tumors are designated by attaching the suffix—*oma* to the cell of origin. For example, a benign tumor arising from fibroblastic cells is called a fibroma, a cartilaginous tumor is a chondroma.

Adenoma is the term applied to a benign epithelial neoplasm that forms glandular patterns as well as tumors derived from glands (Fig. 2.1). Benign epithelial neoplasms producing microscopically or macroscopically visible finger-like or warty projections from epithelial surfaces are referred to as papillomas.

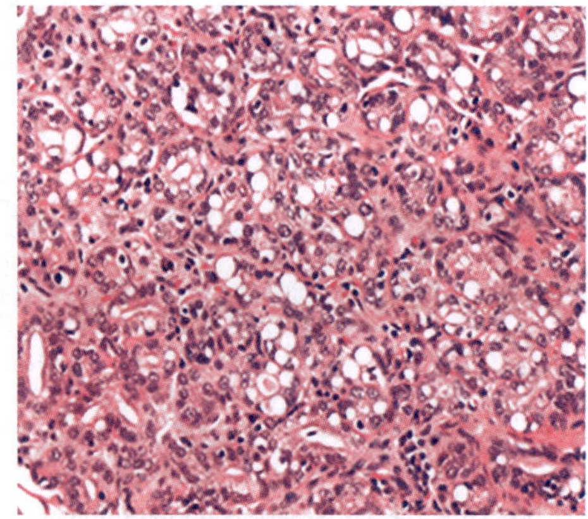

FIGURE 2.1 Adenoma

When a neoplasm, benign or malignant, produces a macroscopically visible projection above a mucosal surface, it is termed a polyp.

Malignant tumors arising in mesenchymal tissue are usually called sarcomas (In Greek *sar* = fleshy), e.g. fibrosarcoma, liposarcoma. Malignant neoplasms of epithelial origin, derived from any of the three germ layers, are called carcinomas. One with glandular pattern microscopically is termed an adenocarcinoma (Fig. 2.2). One producing recognizable squamous cells is termed a squamous cell carcinoma (Fig. 2.3).

Divergent differentiation of a single line of parenchymal cells into another tissue creates

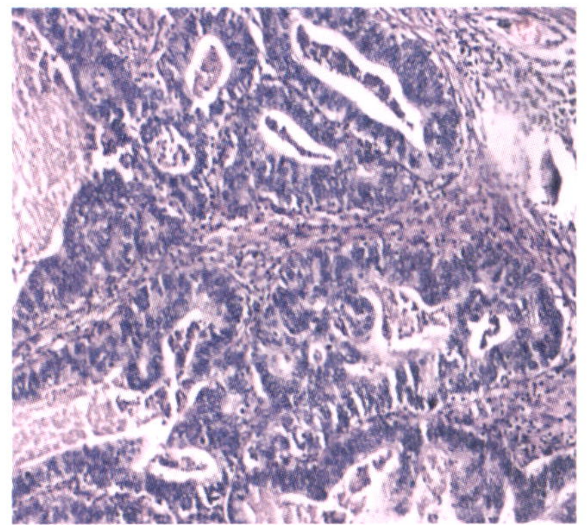

FIGURE 2.2 Adenocarcinoma

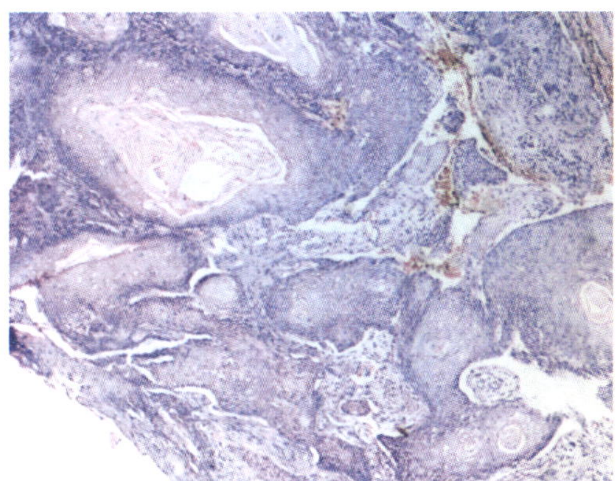

FIGURE 2.3 Squamous cell carcinoma

mixed tumors, e.g. pleomorphic adenoma. Teratomas, are made up of a variety of parenchymal cell types representative of more than one germ layer, usually all three, e.g. ovarian cystic teratoma. Differences between benign and malignant tumors based on their characteristics is given in Table 2.1

HISTORY OF MALIGNANT TUMORS

It has four phases:

1. Malignant change in the target cell referred to as transformation.
2. Growth of transformed cells.
3. Local invasion.
4. Distant metastases.

TABLE 2.1 Classification criteria

Characteristics	*Benign tumor*	*Malignant tumor*
Growth pattern	Cohesive and expansile	Infiltrative
Rate of growth	Slow	Fast
Differentiation	Well	Poor
Metastasis	Absent	Present

DIFFERENTIATION AND ANAPLASIA

Differentiation refers to the extent to which neoplastic cells resemble comparable normal cells, both morphologically and functionally.

Anaplasia is lack of differentiation which is a hallmark of malignant transformation.

Morphological Changes in a Malignant Tumor

- *Pleomorphism*: Variation in the size and shape of cells and the nuclei.
- *Abnormal nuclear morphology:* Nuclei of the tumor cells are larger, hyperchromatic with irregular nuclear membrane. The chromatin is coarsely clumped. The nuclei have prominent nucleoli.
- *Mitoses*: Increased in number and is atypical (Fig. 2.4).
- *Loss of polarity:* The orientation of anaplastic cells is markedly disturbed (i.e. they lose normal polarity). Sheets or large masses of tumor cells grow in an anarchic, disorganized fashion.
- *Other changes:* Tumor giant cells and ischemic necrosis (Fig. 2.5).

DYSPLASIA

Dysplasia means disordered growth. It is characterized by a loss in the uniformity of the individual cells as well as in their architectural orientation. Dysplastic cells exhibit pleomorphism, hyperchromatic nuclei,

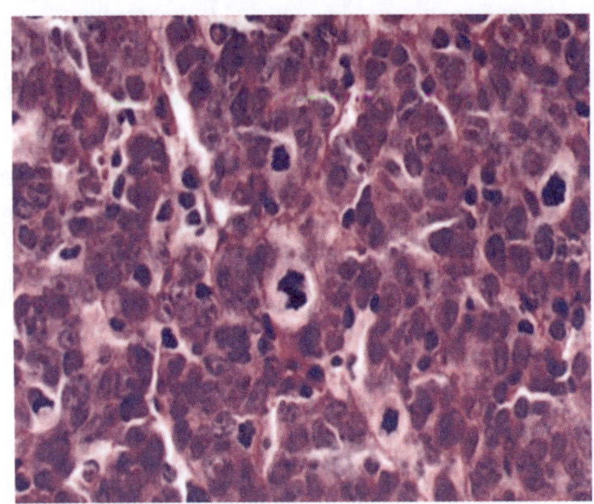

FIGURE 2.4 Atypical mitotic cell

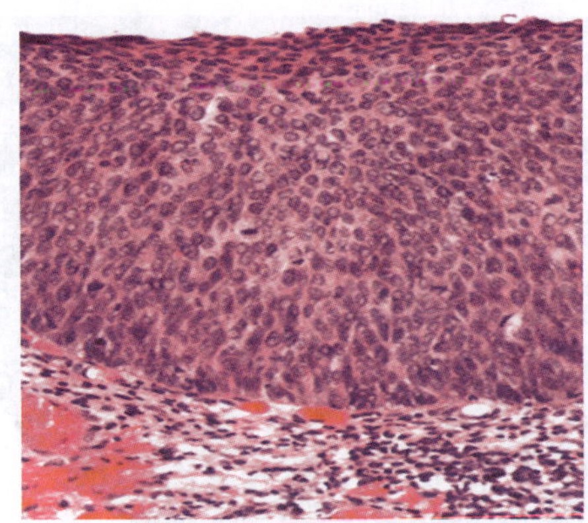

FIGURE 2.6 Carcinoma *in situ*

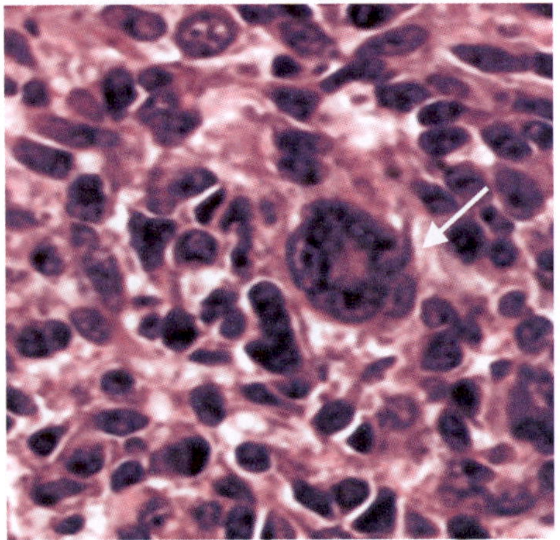

FIGURE 2.5 Tumor giant cell

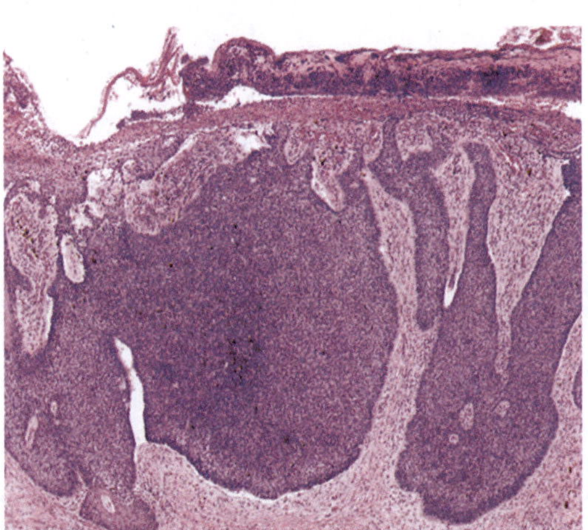

FIGURE 2.7 Basal cell carcinoma showing invasion

abundant mitotic figures, mitoses in abnormal locations within the epithelium.

When dysplastic changes are marked and involve the entire thickness of epithelium, the lesion remains confined to the normal tissue and the basement membrane is intact, it is called carcinoma *in situ*, a preinvasive neoplasm (Fig. 2.6).

INVASION

Nearly all benign tumors grow as cohesive expansile masses that remain localized to their site of origin. They develop a rim of compressed connective tissue, sometimes called a fibrous capsule which separates them from host tissue. But the growth of malignant tumors is accompanied by progressive infiltration, invasion and destruction of surrounding tissue (Fig. 2.7).

Next to metastases, invasiveness is the most reliable feature that differentiates malignant from benign tumors.

METASTASIS

Metastases are tumor implants discontinuous with the primary tumor.

If the tumors are more aggressive, more rapidly growing, and larger in size, greater the likelihood that it will metastasize.

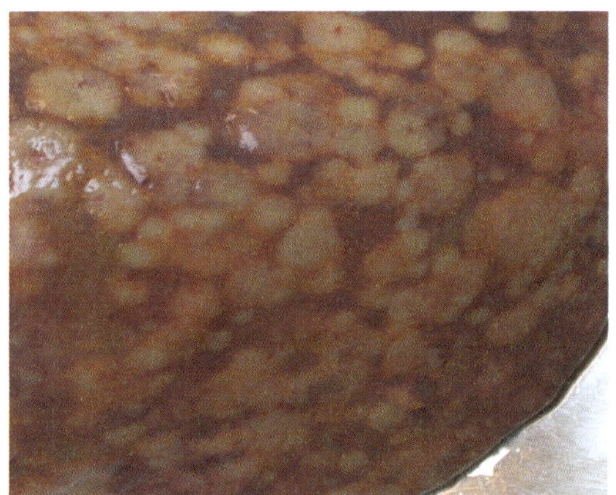

FIGURE 2.8 Metastasis to the liver

PATHWAYS OF SPREAD

- Direct seeding of body cavities or surfaces, e.g. pseudomyxoma peritonei.
- Lymphatic spread is most common for carcinomas and it follows the natural routes of drainage.

  Sentinel lymph node is the first node in a regional lymphatic basin that receives lymph from primary tumor (In breast-axillary lymph node—sentinel lymph node).
- Hematogenous spread is typical for sarcomas but also seen with carcinomas. Liver and lungs are most frequently involved (Fig. 2.8).

CHAPTER 3

Disturbances in the Fluid and Electrolyte Balance

Water is the single most abundant compound in the body, constituting approximately 50 to 70 percent of body weight. Males contain relatively more water (on an average 60%) than females (on an average 50%). There is an inverse relationship between total body fat and total body water (TBW).

The TBW is distributed into two main compartments namely intracellular and extracellular compartments. One-third of body water is extracellular, representing approximately 20 percent of body weight. Of this one-third is located within the intravascular compartment, and two-third is extravascular or interstitial (Fig. 3.1).

Electrolytes are characterized by their degree of dissociation (strong or weak ions). Sodium (Na^+) and chloride (Cl^-) are principally extracellular. Potassium, phosphate, magnesium, and calcium are principally intracellular.

The solute or particle concentration of a fluid is known as its osmolality and is expressed as milliosmoles per kilogram of water (mOsmol/kg). Water crosses cell membranes to achieve osmotic equilibrium (ECF* osmolality = ICF* osmolality). The major ECF particles are Na^+ and its accompanying anions Cl^- and HCO_3^-, whereas K^+ and organic phosphate esters (*ATP, creatine phosphate, and phospholipids) are the predominant ICF osmoles. Solutes that are restricted to the ECF or the ICF determine the effective osmolality (or tonicity) of that compartment. Since Na^+ is largely restricted to the extracellular compartment, total body Na^+

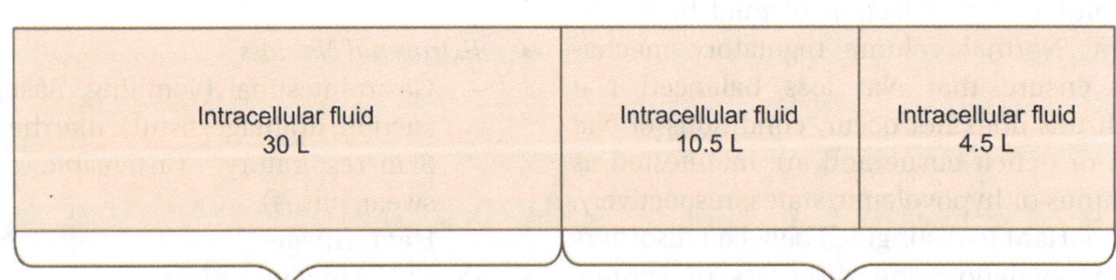

FIGURE 3.1 Major body fluid compartments in a 75 kg male

*ECG = Extracellular fluid
*ICF = Intracellular fluid
*ATP = Adenosine triphosphate

content is a reflection of ECF volume. Likewise, K^+ and its attendant anions are predominantly limited to the ICF and are necessary for normal cell function.

WATER BALANCE

The normal plasma osmolality is 275–290 mOsmol/kg and is kept within a narrow range. To maintain a steady state, water intake must equal water excretion. Disorders of water homeostasis result in hypo- or hypernatremia. Normal individuals have an obligate water loss consisting of urine, stool, and evaporation from the skin and respiratory tract. Gastrointestinal excretion is usually a minor component of total water output, except in patients with vomiting, diarrhea, or high enterostomy output states. Evaporative or insensitive water losses are important in the regulation of core body temperature. Obligatory renal water loss is mandated by the minimum solute excretion required to maintain a steady state. Normally, about 600 mOsmol must be excreted per day, and since the maximal urine osmolality is 1200 mOsmol/kg, a minimum urine output of 500 mL/day is required for neutral solute balance.

SODIUM BALANCE

Sodium is actively pumped out of cells by the Na^+, K^+-ATPase pump. As a result, 85 to 90 percent of all Na^+ is extracellular, and the ECF volume is a reflection of total body Na^+ content. Normal volume regulatory mechanisms ensure that Na^+ loss balanced Na^+ gain. If this does not occur, conditions of Na^+ excess or deficit ensue and are manifested as edematous or hypovolemic states, respectively. It is important to distinguish between disorders of osmoregulation and disorders of volume regulation since water and Na^+ balance are regulated independently. Changes in Na^+ concentration generally reflect disturbed water homeostasis, whereas alterations in Na^+ content are manifested as ECF volume contraction or expansion and imply abnormal Na^+ balance.

POTASSIUM BALANCE

Potassium is the major intracellular cation. The normal plasma K^+ concentration is 3.5 to 5.0 mmol/L, whereas that inside cells is about 150 mmol/L. Therefore, the amount of K^+ in the ECF (30–70 mmol) constitutes less than two percent of the total body K^+ content (2500–4500 mmol). The ratio of ICF to ECF K^+ concentration (normally 38:1) is the principal result of the resting membrane potential and is crucial for normal neuromuscular function. The basolateral Na^+, K^+-ATPase pump actively transports K^+ in and Na^+ out of the cell in a 2:3 ratio, and the passive outward diffusion of K^+ is quantitatively the most important factor that generates the resting membrane potential. The activity of the electrogenic Na^+, K^+-ATPase pump may be stimulated as a result of an increased intracellular Na^+ concentration and inhibited in the setting of digoxin toxicity or chronic illness such as heart failure or renal failure.

HYPOVOLEMIA

True volume depletion, or hypovolemia, generally refers to a state of combined salt and water loss exceeding intake, leading to ECF volume contraction. The loss of Na^+ may be renal or extrarenal.

Causes of Hypovolemia

ECF Volume Contracted

- *Extrarenal Na^+ loss*
  - Gastrointestinal (vomiting, nasogastric suction, drainage, fistula, diarrhea)
  - Skin/respiratory (insensible losses, sweat, burns)
  - Hemorrhage
- *Renal Na^+ and water loss*
  - Diuretics
  - Osmotic diuresis
  - Hypoaldosteronism
  - Salt-wasting nephropathies
- *Renal water loss:* Diabetes insipidus (central or nephrogenic).

ECF Volume Normal or Expanded

- *Decreased cardiac output:* Myocardial, valvular, or pericardial disease
- *Redistribution*
  - Hypoalbuminemia (hepatic cirrhosis, nephrotic syndrome)
  - Capillary leak (acute pancreatitis, ischemic bowel, rhabdomyolysis)
- *Increased venous capacitance:* Sepsis.

Clinical Features

Most symptoms are nonspecific and secondary to electrolyte imbalances and tissue hypoperfusion and include fatigue, weakness, muscle cramps, thirst, and postural dizziness. More severe degrees of volume contraction can lead to end-organ ischemia which manifested as oliguria, cyanosis, abdominal and chest pain, and confusion or obtundation. Diminished skin turgor and dry oral mucous membranes are poor markers of decreased interstitial fluid.

Signs of intravascular volume contraction include decreased jugular venous pressure, postural hypotension, and postural tachycardia. Larger and more acute fluid losses lead to hypovolemic shock, manifested as hypotension, tachycardia, peripheral vasoconstriction, and hypoperfusion—cyanosis, cold and clammy extremities, oliguria, and altered mental status.

HYPONATREMIA

A plasma Na^+ concentration <135 mmol/L usually reflects a hypotonic state.

Causes of Hyponatremia

Pseudohyponatremia

- *Normal plasma osmolality*
  - Hyperlipidemia
  - Hyperproteinemia
  - Post-transurethral resection of prostate/bladder tumor
- *Increased plasma osmolality*
  - Hyperglycemia
  - Mannitol.

Hypo-osmolar Hyponatremia

- *Primary Na^+ loss (secondary water gain)*
  - *Integumentary loss:* Sweating, burns
  - *Gastrointestinal loss:* Vomiting, tube drainage, fistula, obstruction, diarrhea
  - *Renal loss:* Diuretics, osmotic diuresis, hypoaldosteronism, salt-wasting nephropathy, postobstructive diuresis, nonoliguric acute tubular necrosis
- *Primary water gain (secondary Na^+ loss)*
  - Primary polydipsia
  - Decreased solute intake (e.g. beer potomania)
  - AVP* release due to pain, nausea, drugs
  - Syndrome of inappropriate AVP* secretion
  - Glucocorticoid deficiency
  - Hypothyroidism
  - Chronic renal insufficiency
- *Primary Na^+ gain (exceeded by secondary water gain)*
  - Heart failure
  - Hepatic cirrhosis
  - Nephrotic syndrome.

Clinical Features

The clinical manifestations of hyponatremia are related to specifically brain cell swelling or cerebral edema. Therefore, the symptoms are primarily neurologic, and their severity is dependent on the rapidity of onset and absolute decrease in plasma Na^+ concentration. Patients may be asymptomatic or complain of nausea and malaise. As the plasma Na^+ concentration falls, the symptoms progress to include headache, lethargy, confusion, and obtundation. Stupor, seizures, and coma do not usually occur, unless the plasma Na^+ concentration falls acutely below 120 mmol/L or decreases rapidly.

HYPERNATREMIA

Hypernatremia is defined as a plasma Na^+ concentration >145 mmol/L. Hypernatremia

*AVP = Arginine vasopressin

may be due to primary Na^+ gain or water deficit. The two components of an appropriate response to hypernatremia are increased water intake stimulated by thirst and the excretion of the minimum volume of maximally concentrated urine.

The source of free water loss is either renal or extrarenal. Nonrenal loss of water may be due to evaporation from the skin and respiratory tract (insensible losses) or loss from the gastrointestinal tract. Insensible losses are increased with fever, exercise, heat exposure, and severe burns and in mechanically ventilated patients. Furthermore, the Na^+ concentration of sweat decreases with profuse perspiration, thereby increasing solute-free water loss. Diarrhea is the most common gastrointestinal cause of hypernatremia. Specifically, osmotic diarrheas (induced by lactulose, sorbitol, or malabsorption of carbohydrate) and viral gastroenteritides result in water loss, exceeding that of Na^+ and K^+.

Renal water loss is the most common cause of hypernatremia and is due to drug-induced or osmotic diuresis or diabetes insipidus. Hypernatremia secondary to nonosmotic urinary water loss is usually due to: (1) Central diabetes insipidus (CDI) or (2) Nephrogenic diabetes insipidus (NDI) resulting from end organ (renal).

Clinical Features

The major symptoms of hypernatremia are neurologic and include altered mental status, weakness, neuromuscular irritability, focal neurologic deficits, and occasionally coma or seizures. Patients may also complain of polyuria or thirst. For unknown reasons, patients with polydipsia from CDI tend to prefer ice-cold water.

HYPOKALEMIA

Hypokalemia, defined as a plasma K^+ concentration <3.5 mmol/L, may result from one (or more) of the following: Decreased net intake, shift into cells or increased net loss.

Causes of Hypokalemia

Decreased Intake

- Starvation
- Clay ingestion

Redistribution into Cells

- *Acid-base*
  - Metabolic alkalosis
- *Hormonal*
  - Insulin
  - Adrenergic agonists (endogenous or exogenous)
  - Adrenergic antagonists
- *Anabolic state*
  - Vitamin B_{12} or folic acid (red blood cell production)
  - Granulocyte-macrophage colony stimulating factor (white blood cell production)
  - Total parenteral nutrition
- *Other*
  - Pseudohypokalemia
  - Hypothermia
  - Hypokalemic periodic paralysis
  - Barium toxicity.

Increased Loss

- *Nonrenal*
  - Gastrointestinal loss (diarrhea)
  - Integumentary loss (sweat)
- *Renal*
  - *Increased distal flow*: Diuretics, osmotic diuresis, salt-wasting nephropathies
  - Increased secretion of potassium
    - *Mineralocorticoid excess:* Primary hyperaldosteronism, secondary hyperaldosteronism (malignant hypertension, renin-secreting tumors, renal artery stenosis, hypovolemia), apparent mineralocorticoid excess (licorice, chewing tobacco, carbenoxolone), congenital adrenal hyperplasia, Cushing's syndrome, Bartter's syndrome
    - *Distal delivery of nonreabsorbed anions:* Vomiting, nasogastric

suction, proximal (type 2) renal tubular acidosis, diabetic ketoacidosis, glue-sniffing (toluene abuse), penicillin derivatives

- *Others:* Amphotericin B, Liddle's syndrome, hypomagnesemia.

Clinical Features

The clinical manifestations of K^+ depletion vary greatly between individual patients, and their severity depends on the degree of hypokalemia. Symptoms seldom occur unless the plasma K^+ concentration is <3 mmol/L. Fatigue, myalgia, and muscular weakness of the lower extremities are common complaints and are due to a lower (more negative) resting membrane potential. More severe hypokalemia may lead to progressive weakness, hypoventilation (due to respiratory muscle involvement), and eventually complete paralysis. Impaired muscle metabolism and the blunted hyperemic response to exercise associated with profound K^+ depletion increase the risk of rhabdomyolysis. Smooth-muscle function may also be affected and manifested as paralytic ileus.

HYPERKALEMIA

Hyperkalemia, defined as a plasma K^+ concentration >5.0 mmol/L, occurs as a result of either K^+ release from cells or decreased renal loss. Increased K^+ intake is rarely the sole cause of hyperkalemia, since the phenomenon of potassium adaptation ensures rapid K^+ excretion in response to increases in dietary consumption. Iatrogenic hyperkalemia may result from overzealous parenteral K^+ replacement or in patients with renal insufficiency. Pseudohyperkalemia represents an artificially elevated plasma K^+ concentration due to K^+ movement out of cells immediately prior to or following venipuncture. Contributing factors include prolonged use of a tourniquet with or without repeated fist clenching, hemolysis, and marked leukocytosis or thrombocytosis. The latter two result in an elevated serum K^+ concentration due to release of intracellular K^+ following clot formation. Pseudohyperkalemia should be suspected in an otherwise asymptomatic patient with no obvious underlying cause. If proper venipuncture technique is used and a plasma (not serum) K^+ concentration is measured, it should be normal. Intravascular hemolysis, tumor lysis syndrome, and rhabdomyolysis all lead to K^+ release from cells as a result of tissue breakdown.

Causes of Hyperkalemia

- Renal failure
- Decreased distal flow (i.e. decreased effective circulating arterial volume)
- Decreased K^+ secretion

Impaired Na^+ reabsorption

- *Primary hypoaldosteronism:* Adrenal insufficiency, adrenal enzyme deficiency (21-hydroxylase, 3-hydroxysteroid dehydrogenase, corticosterone methyl oxidase)
- *Secondary hypoaldosteronism:* Hyporeninemia, drugs (*ACE inhibitors, *NSAIDs, heparin)
- *Resistance to aldosterone:* Pseudohypoaldosteronism, tubulointerstitial disease, drugs (K^+-sparing diuretics, trimethoprim, pentamidine)

Enhanced Cl^- reabsorption (chloride shunt)

- Gordon's syndrome
- Cyclosporine.

Clinical Features

Since the resting membrane potential is related to the ratio of the ICF to ECF K^+ concentration, hyperkalemia partially depolarizes the cell membrane. Prolonged depolarization impairs membrane excitability and is manifested as weakness, which may progress to flaccid paralysis and hypoventilation, if the respiratory muscles are involved. The most serious effect of hyperkalemia is cardiac toxicity, which does not correlate well with the plasma K^+ concentration.

*ACE = Angiotensin-converting enzyme
*NSAIDs = Nonsteroidal anti-inflammatory drugs

CHAPTER 4

Respiratory System

ANATOMY

The respiratory system consists of the trachea, bronchial tree and the lungs. The right and the left main bronchi divide into smaller bronchioles which further divide to form terminal bronchiole. The part of the lung distal to the terminal bronchiole is called an acinus. An acinus consists of respiratory bronchiole (distal to the terminal bronchiole) and alveoli. The alveolus consists of alveolar ducts and alveolar sacs. The gas exchange takes place at the level of the alveoli (Fig. 4.1).

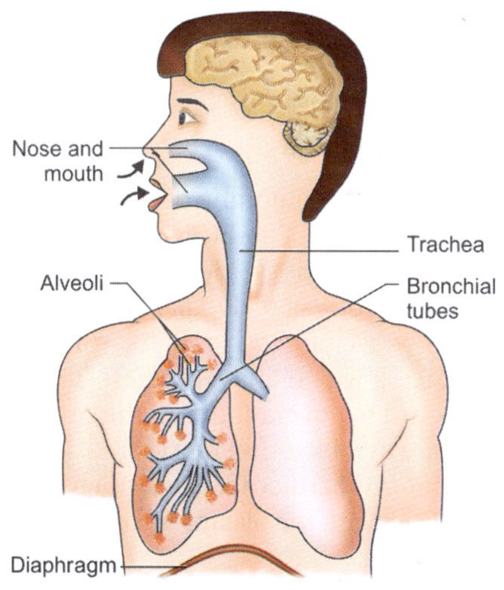

FIGURE 4.1 Anatomy of respiratory system

HISTOLOGY

The bronchial tree is lined by the pseudostratified ciliated columnar epithelium admixed with cartilage and mucin secreting goblet cells. The microscopic picture of lung consists of empty alveolar spaces (as they are filled with air normally) and the pulmonary interstitium. The alveolar spaces are lined by alveolar cells (type I and type II pneumocytes) and the interstitium consisting of fine elastic fibers, few collagen fibers, fibroblasts and smooth muscle cells.

PULMONARY TUBERCULOSIS

Tuberculosis is caused by the bacterium *Mycobacterium tuberculosis*. The mode of transmission is by aerosol spread from person-to-person.

Epidemiologically, tuberculosis is rampant in India with a high rate of incidence and prevalence. There has been a sudden increase in the number of tuberculosis cases due to its association with HIV.

In *M. tuberculosis*, it is important that we differentiate between infection and disease. Infection is the presence of organisms, which may or may not cause clinically significant disease. Most infections are acquired by person-to-person transmission of airborne droplets of organisms from an active case to a susceptible host.

Infection with *M. tuberculosis* typically leads to the development of delayed hypersensitivity to *M. tuberculosis* antigens, which can be detected by the tuberculin (Mantoux) test. A positive tuberculin test indicates cell mediated hypersensitivity to tubercular antigens.

Clinical Features of Tuberculosis

There are four clinicopathological forms of tuberculosis:

1. Primary tuberculosis
2. Progressive primary tuberculosis
3. Secondary tuberculosis
4. Miliary tuberculosis.

Primary Tuberculosis

Primary tuberculosis is the form of the disease that develops in a previously unexposed, unsensitized person. Clinically significant symptoms develop in about 5 percent of newly infected people. The source of infection is exogenous from an active case of tuberculosis.

Most of the patients with primary tuberculosis go into a latent phase. But some cases progress with continued lung disease and are called progressive primary tuberculosis. These patients usually present with lower and middle lung lobe consolidation and hilar lymphadenopathy.

Secondary Tuberculosis

Secondary tuberculosis is a pattern that arises in a previously sensitized host. It may follow shortly after primary infection, but usually arises due to reactivation of latent primary infection after many years. Reactivation occurs when the host immunity is reduced. Secondary pulmonary tuberculosis classically involves the apex of the upper lobes of one or both lungs. It will lead to cavitation of lung.

Morphology

Primary Tuberculosis

In primary pulmonary tuberculosis, the inhaled bacilli implant in the distal airspaces close to the pleura. This leads to the development of a gray-white inflammatory consolidated area measuring 1–1.5 cm. This is known as **Ghon focus**. The center of this focus undergoes caseous necrosis. The tubercle bacilli will then infect the draining lymph nodes which also caseate. This combination of parenchymal lung lesion and nodal involvement is known as Ghon complex (Figs 4.2 and 4.3).

Microscopically the hallmark of active disease is characterized by the development of **caseating granulomatous inflammation** that forms tubercles. The granuloma is characterized by central caseation necrosis, modified macrophages called epithelioid cells, Langhans giant cells (Large cell with multiple nuclei arranged at one pole of the cell in the form of horse shoe), rimmed by lymphocytes and fibroblasts (Fig. 4.4).

Secondary Tuberculosis

The initial lesion is usually a small focus of consolidation less than 2 cm in diameter and located within 1 to 2 cm of the apical pleura, grossly they are sharply defined gray-white areas. Microscopically, they are characterized by caseating granulomas.

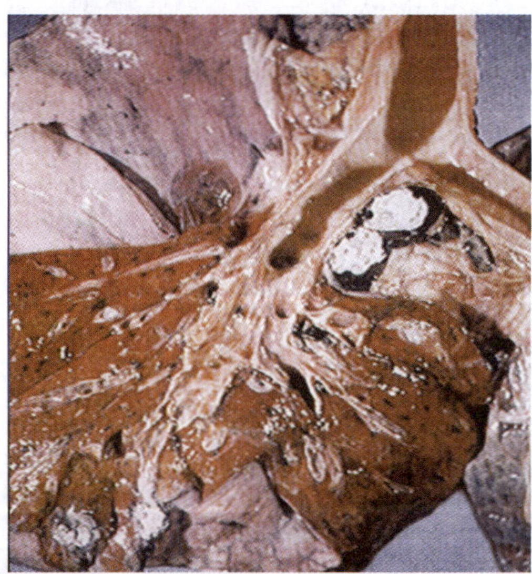

FIGURE 4.2 Note the Ghon complex

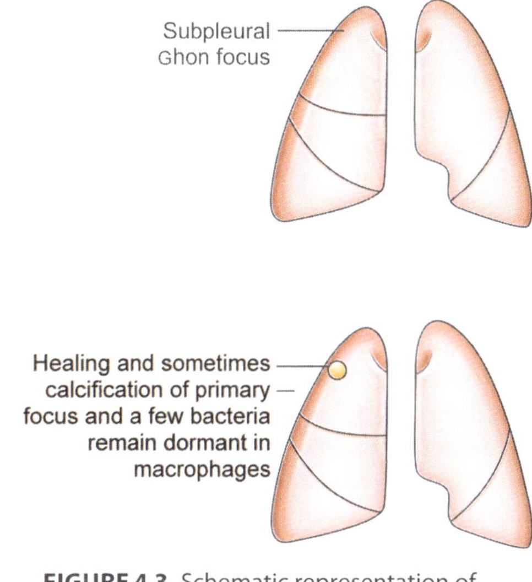

FIGURE 4.3 Schematic representation of Ghon's focus

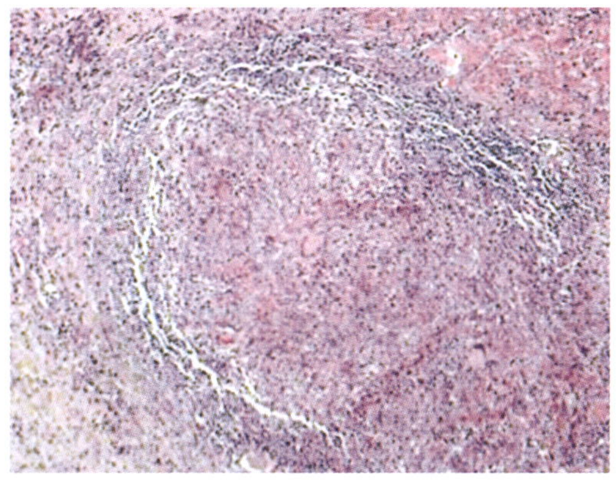

FIGURE 4.4 Microscopic view of caseating granuloma

Progressive primary tuberculosis may be seen in the elderly and in the immunocompromised. The apical lesion enlarges with the expansion of central caseation area. This erodes into the bronchus creating an irregular cavity. This is called cavitary pulmonary tuberculosis. Erosion of the blood vessel leads to blood mixed sputum (hemoptysis) (Fig. 4.5).

Miliary pulmonary tuberculosis develops when organisms drain through lymphatics into

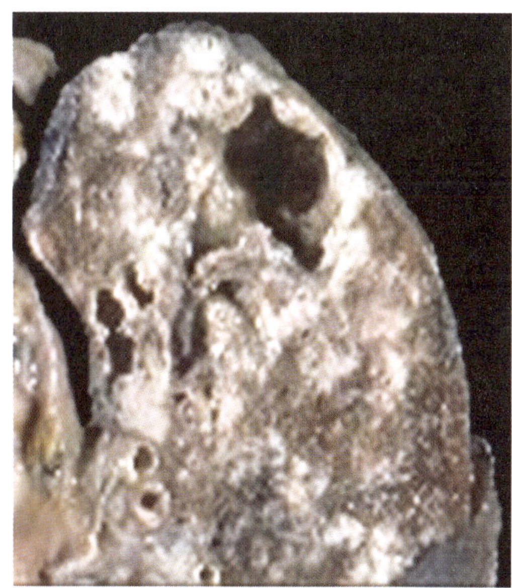

FIGURE 4.5 Gross appearance of cavitary tuberculous lung disease

the lymphatic ducts and empty into right side of heart. From here it will drain into the pulmonary arteries and so both the lungs are involved. This result in multiple, small (2 mm) foci of yellow-white consolidation scattered through the lung parenchyma giving the appearance of "millet" seeds. This may later lead to dissemination of the infection throughout the body leading to systemic miliary tuberculosis (Fig. 4.6).

Diagnosis

The diagnosis of pulmonary tuberculosis is based on history, clinical examination, Radiological findings and laboratory investigations. History of fever with evening rise of temperature, cough with sputum for more than 3 months, hemoptysis and weight loss suggest the possibility. Chest X-ray showing cavity and consolidation may point towards the possible diagnosis. Mantoux positive is also a helpful test. But the ultimate evidence is the identification of acid fast bacilli in the sputum. Culture may take 10 weeks to grow (Figs 4.7 and 4.8).

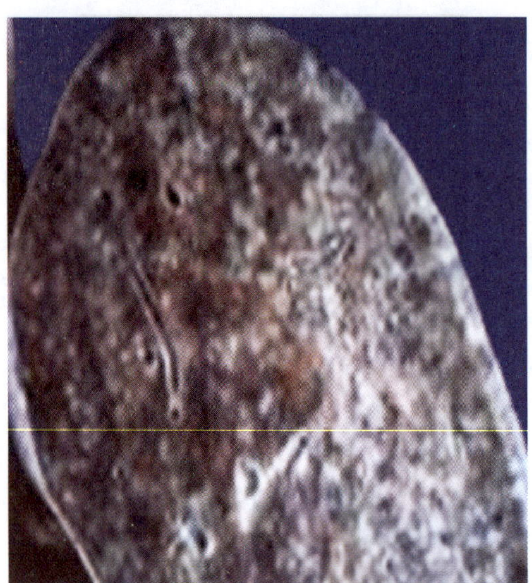

FIGURE 4.6 Gross appearance of miliary tuberculosis

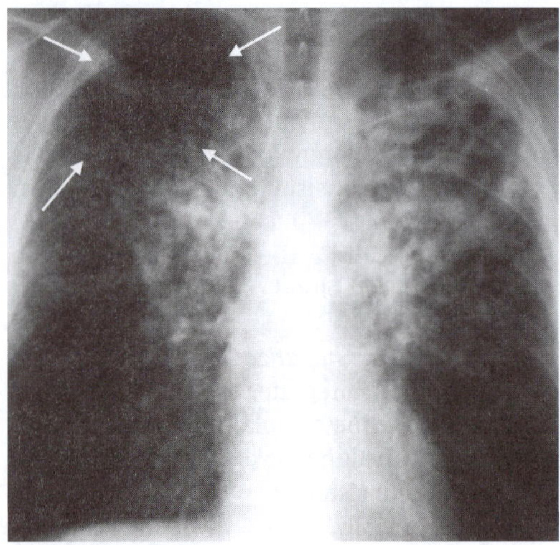

FIGURE 4.7 Chest X-ray with bilateral upper lobe opacities (white areas) with multiple cavities including a very large cavity in the right upper lobe (arrows)

PNEUMONIA

Pneumonia can be defined as the infection of the lung parenchyma.

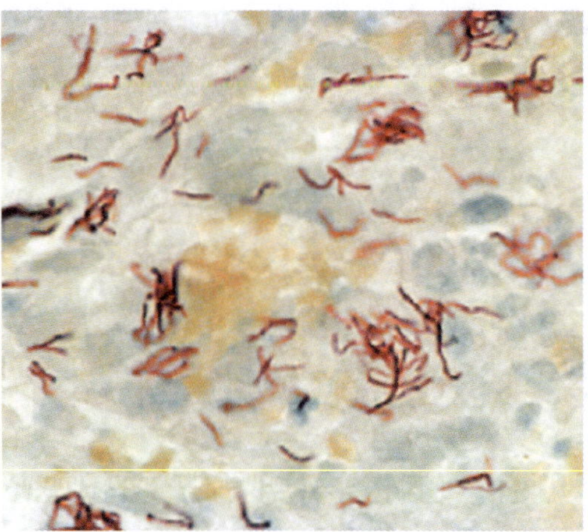

FIGURE 4.8 Sputum showing acid fast bacilli

Etiology

Pneumonia can be caused by a variety of bacterial, viral and fungal organisms. The common offending agents are *Streptococcus pneumoniae, Staphylococcus aureus, Moraxella catarrhalis,* gram negative pathogens, viruses and fungi (*Candida* and *Aspergillus*).

Factors predisposing to the development of pneumonia:
- Loss of suppression of cough reflex as in coma and anesthesia
- Injury to the mucociliary apparatus as seen in cigarette smokers
- Alcohol, tobacco, smoke will interfere with the activity of alveolar macrophages
- Pulmonary congestion and edema
- Accumulation of secretions.

Classification of Pneumonia

There are two types of classification.
1. Depending on the way it is acquired, it can be classified as:
    - Community-acquired pneumonia
    - Hospital-acquired pneumonia
    - Aspiration pneumonia
    - Chronic pneumonia.
2. Depending on the morphological involvement, it can be classified as:

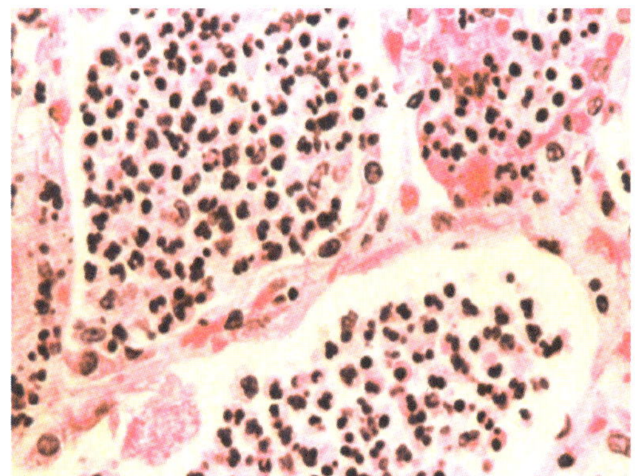

FIGURE 4.9 Microscopic picture of lobar pneumonia

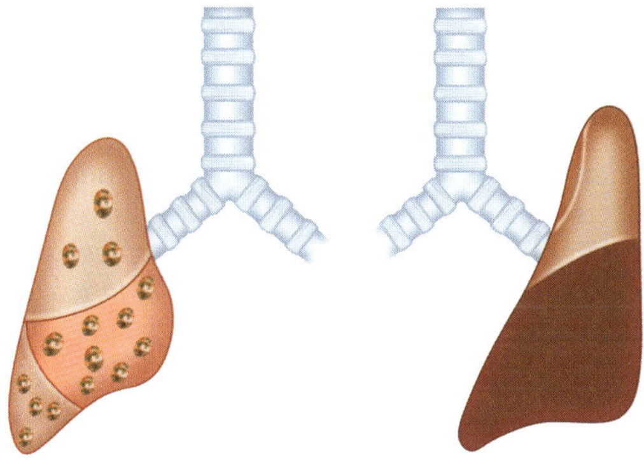

FIGURE 4.10 Schematic representation of the gross involvement of lung in lobar and bronchopneumonia

- Lobar pneumonia
- Bronchopneumonia.

Lobar Pneumonia

It is an acute bacterial infection resulting in fibrinosuppurative consolidation of one entire lobe of the lung (Fig. 4.11).

Classically four stages have been described in lobar pneumonia. All these stages may be masked due to modern day effective antibiotic treatment.

1. *Stage of congestion:* Grossly the lung is heavy, boggy and red due to increased blood flow.
   Microscopically, the alveolar lumen is filled with inflammatory exudate consisting of neutrophils and bacteria.

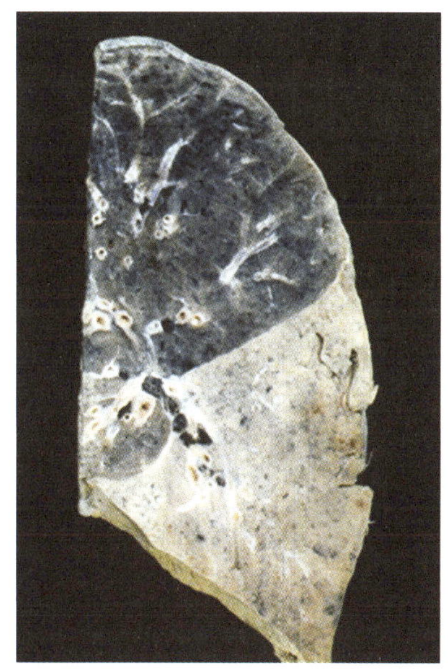

FIGURE 4.11 Gross involvement of one lobe in lobar pneumonia

2. *Stage of red hepatization:* Grossly the lung is heavy, red, firm and airless. Thus, it loses its normal spongy consistency and gets a liver-like consistency, hence the term hepatization.
   Microscopically, the alveolar exudate consists of red blood cells, neutrophils and fibrin.
3. *Stage of gray hepatization:* In this stage, the RBCs disintegrate, the hemosiderin is taken up by the alveolar macrophages and so grossly the lung looks gray in color with a liver-like consistency.
   Microscopically, the alveolar exudate consists of disintegrated RBCs, hemosiderin laden macrophages and fibrin. The fibrin contracts the alveolar exudate so that a clear space is seen between the alveolar septa and the exudate.
4. *Stage of resolution:* The exudate undergoes progressive enzymatic digestion which produces granular debris which is either coughed out or absorbed by the lymphatics (Fig. 4.9).

Bronchopneumonia

It is acute infection of the lung which involves patchy consolidation of the lung (Fig. 4.10).

LUNG ABSCESS

Lung abscess is described as localized suppurative infection of the lung, characterized by necrosis of lung tissue.

Etiology

The most common pathogens causing lung abscess include streptococci, *Staphylococcus*, anaerobic organisms like *Bacteroides, Fusobacterium* and *Peptococcus.*

The mode of entry of the causative organism is as follows:

- Aspiration of infective material in conditions such as coma, anesthesia, debilitation and gingivodental sepsis
- Following bacterial infection of lung (after pneumonia)
- Septic embolism
- Secondary infection following obstruction due to tumors
- Direct penetrating trauma.

Morphology

Abscesses vary in size from few millimeters to large cavities of 5 to 6 cm. They can be single or multiple and affect any part of the lung. The abscess cavity is filled with suppurative debris. The hallmark change in all abscesses is suppurative destruction of lung parenchyma within the central area of cavitation.

Clinical Features

Patients have fever and cough with copious amount of foul smelling purulent sputum production. Chest pain and weight loss can be seen.

Treatment

Antibiotics are the main line of therapy.

BRONCHIECTASIS

Bronchiectasis is a disease characterized by permanent dilatation of bronchi and bronchioles caused by destruction of the muscle and elastic tissue, resulting from or associated with chronic necrotizing infections. To call it bronchiectasis, the dilatation should be permanent.

Etiology

There are two things associated with bronchiectasis—obstruction and infection. Obstruction could be due to impaction of mucus or foreign body or tumors. The normal clearing mechanisms are impaired due to obstruction which results in the pooling of secretions distal to the obstruction and its inflammation.

Conditions associated with bronchiectasis:

1. Congenital or hereditary conditions such as cystic fibrosis, primary ciliary dyskinesia and Kartagener syndromes.
2. Postinfectious conditions such as pneumonia due to bacteria, virus and fungi.
3. Bronchial obstruction due to tumors, foreign body or mucus impaction.

Morphology

Gross

Bronchiectasis usually affects lower lobes bilaterally. The airways are dilated, sometimes up to four times its normal size. Depending on the shape of the bronchial enlargement, it can be divided into three types:

1. *Cylindrical bronchiectasis*: Long tube like dilatations.
2. Fusiform bronchiectasis.
3. Saccular bronchiectasis.

Microscopy

In a full blown case of bronchiectasis, acute and chronic inflammatory exudate is seen in the walls of the bronchi and bronchioles. Also seen

is the desquamation of the lining epithelium and large areas of necrosis and ulceration. In long-standing cases, fibrosis of bronchial and bronchiolar walls develops leading to obliteration of the bronchiolar lumina.

On culture, it usually yields staphylococci, streptococci, pneumococci and anaerobic organisms or fungi such as *Aspergillus*.

Clinical Features

Bronchiectasis presents as severe persistent cough with expectoration of copious foul smelling sputum. Breathlessness and blood tinged sputum can be seen in few cases.

CHRONIC OBSTRUCTIVE PULMONARY DISEASE

Chronic obstructive pulmonary disease (COPD) is a clinical term which refers to two diseases with overlapping symptoms and signs—chronic bronchitis and emphysema. Both these diseases cause chronic obstruction of the airways as a result of long-term heavy cigarette smoking. About 10 percent of these patients are nonsmokers.

EMPHYSEMA/PINK PUFFERS

Emphysema is a condition of the lung characterized by abnormal permanent enlargement of the airspaces distal to the terminal bronchiole accompanied by destruction of their walls and without obvious fibrosis.

Types of Emphysema

Emphysema is classified according to its anatomical distribution within the lobule.

1. *Centriacinar:* This involves the proximal or the central parts of the acini. The respiratory bronchioles are affected but distal alveoli are spared. This type occurs predominantly in heavy smokers and in association with chronic bronchitis.
2. *Panacinar*: This involves the acini uniformly from the level of respiratory bronchiole to the terminal blind alveoli.
3. *Paraseptal (Distal acinar)*: In this type only the distal part of the acinus is involved but the proximal part is normal.
4. *Irregular:* It is so named because the acinus is irregularly involved (Fig. 4.12).

Morphology

Gross

In panacinar emphysema, the lungs are large, overlapping the heart. In irregular emphysema, apical blebs and bullae are characteristic (Fig. 4.13).

Microscopy

Abnormally large alveoli separated by thin septa with only focal centriacinar fibrosis (Fig. 4.14).

Clinical Features

Dyspnea or breathlessness is slowly progressive. Cough may or may not be present. Weight loss is a prominent symptom. Classically, the patient is barrel chested and dyspneic, with prolonged expiration, sits forward in a hunched position and breathes through pursed lips as if puffing. They do not have cyanosis. So, they are referred to as pink puffers.

CHRONIC BRONCHITIS

Chronic bronchitis is defined as persistent cough with sputum production for at least 3 months in at least 2 consecutive years, in absence of any identifiable cause.

Etiology

The primary initiating factor in the genesis of chronic bronchitis is chronic irritation caused by inhaled substances such as tobacco smoke (90% of patients are smokers) and grain, cotton and silica dust. Bacterial and viral infections are

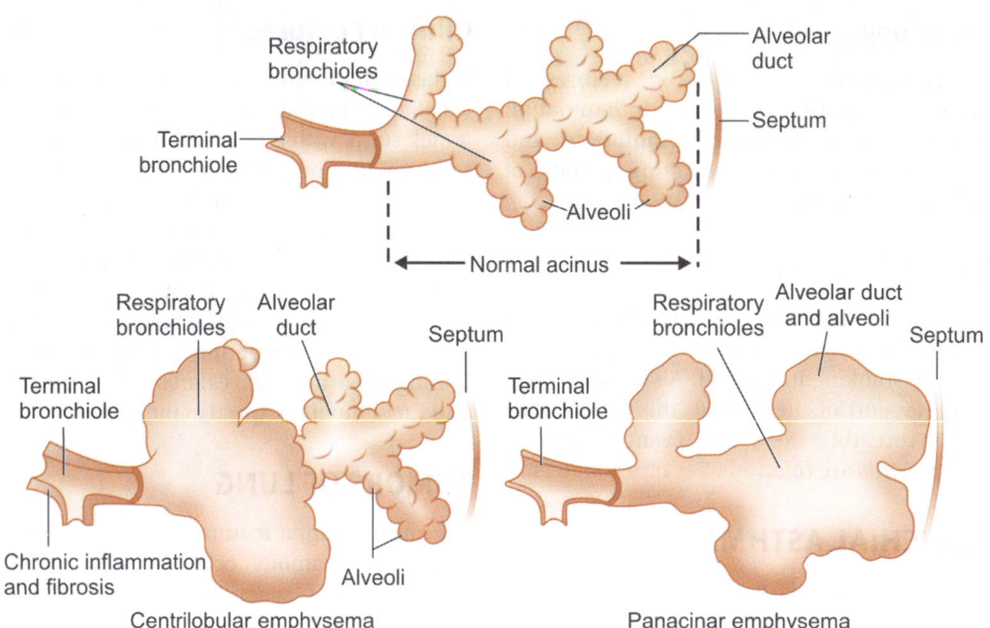

FIGURE 4.12 Schematic representation of types of emphysema

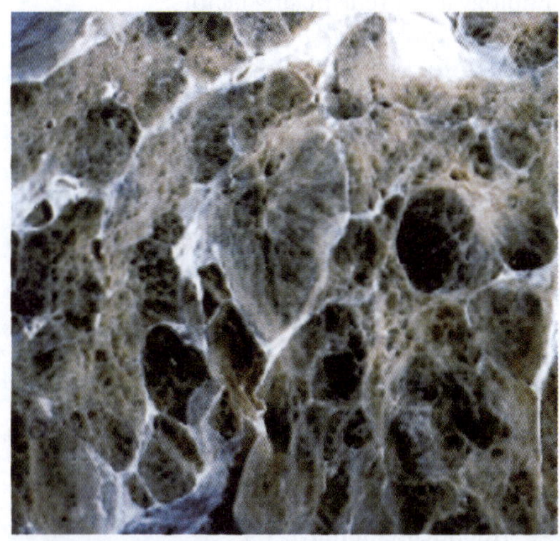

FIGURE 4.13 Gross appearance of emphysema showing markedly enlarged air spaces

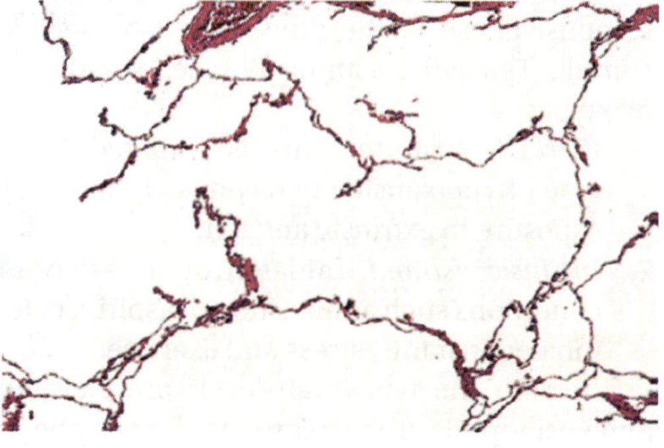

FIGURE 4.14 Microscopy of emphysema showing large irregular air spaces

important triggers in the exacerbation of the disease. Chronic bronchitis is most frequently seen in middle aged men. It is 4 to 10 times more common in smokers.

Morphology

Gross

There may be hyperemia, congestion, swelling and edema of the mucous membranes associated with excessive mucinous and mucopurulent secretions layering the epithelial surfaces.

Microscopy

The characteristic microscopic features of chronic bronchitis are chronic inflammation of airways with lymphocytic infiltrate and enlargement of mucus secreting glands of trachea and bronchi.

Clinical Features

The hallmark symptom of chronic bronchitis is a persistent cough with sputum production in a heavily smoking individual. After many years of progression of the disease the patient may develop breathlessness and cyanosis and so these patients are referred to as blue bloaters.

BRONCHIAL ASTHMA

Bronchial asthma is a chronic inflammatory disorder of the airways that causes recurrent episodes of wheezing, breathlessness, chest tightness and cough, particularly at night and/ or early morning.

Asthma is usually caused by increased responsiveness of the airways to a variety of stimuli. Typically, asthma is categorized into two types:

1. *Extrinsic asthma*: This is initiated by a type I hypersensitivity response induced by exposure to extrinsic antigen.
2. *Intrinsic asthma*: Initiated by a variety of conditions such as ingestion of aspirin, cold, inhaled irritants, stress and exercise.

In both the types, IgE levels are elevated and eosinophils are increased in the peripheral blood.

Morphology

Lungs are overdistended. The most important features are presence of thick tenacious mucous plugs occluding the bronchi and Curschmann's spirals (mucous plugs containing shed epithelium).

Clinical Features

A classical presentation of symptoms in asthma is called as an asthmatic attack. Typically each attack starts with a bout of cough with sputum production along with difficulty in breathing and lasts up to several hours. These attacks are more common in the night or in the early mornings and are triggered by cold, stress, pollen, etc. The clinical diagnosis is helped by the demonstration of an increased number of eosinophils in the peripheral blood, and the finding of eosinophils, Charcot Leyden crystals and Curschmann's spiral in the sputum.

TUMORS OF LUNG

The most important tumors that occur in the lung are squamous cell carcinoma, adeno-carcinoma and secondary metastasis to the lung.

Lung Cancer

Etiology and predisposing factors:

- *Tobacco smoking:* Average smokers have a 10-fold increased risk of developing lung cancer than nonsmokers. It depends on the duration of smoking and the amount of cigarettes smoked per day.
- *Industrial hazards:* Increased incidence of lung cancer is seen in people exposed to ionizing radiation, radioactive element uranium and exposure to asbestos.

Classification

Histologic classification of lung tumors is as follows:

- Squamous cell carcinoma
- Adenocarcinoma
- Small cell carcinoma
- Large cell carcinoma.

Lung cancer has a peak age incidence at 50 to 60 years.

Morphology

Squamous Cell Carcinoma

This is usually seen in heavy smokers. It begins as a small focus and can grow as large cauliflower like fungating mass filling the bronchi and extending into the mediastinum. Microscopically, the tumor cells are round to polygonal with abundant eosinophilic cytoplasm, large nucleus and a prominent nucleolus; keratin pearls and individual cell keratinization can be seen. Mitotic figures can also be present (Fig. 4.15).

The squamous cell carcinoma (SCC) spreads through blood and lymphatics.

Adenocarcinoma

It is seen commonly in women and non-smokers. It can grow as papillary fronds located more commonly at the periphery of the lung. Microscopically, it is characterized by glandular differentiation or mucin production of the tumor cells (Fig. 4.16).

Small Cell Carcinoma

This is a highly malignant tumor. Microscopically, it is characterized by small cells with scanty cytoplasm finely granular salt and pepper nuclear chromatin and absent nucleolus.

Large Cell Carcinoma

This is an undifferentiated type of tumor which has large cells with moderate amount of cytoplasm, large nucleus and prominent nucleolus.

Clinical Features

Majority of the patients are in their fifties, with symptoms of cough, weight loss, chest pain and dyspnea. The prognosis of these is poor. Even with improved techniques of surgery, radiotherapy and chemotherapy the 5-year survival is 15 percent.

PLEURA

Pleural Effusion

Pleural effusion is a common manifestation of both primary and secondary pleural diseases (Table 4.1). Normally about 15 mL of serous, relatively acellular, clear fluid lubricates the pleural surface. Increased accumulation of pleural fluid occurs in the following conditions:

- Increased hydrostatic pressure as in congestive heart failure.
- Increased vascular permeability as in pneumonia.
- Decreased osmotic pressure as in nephrotic syndrome.

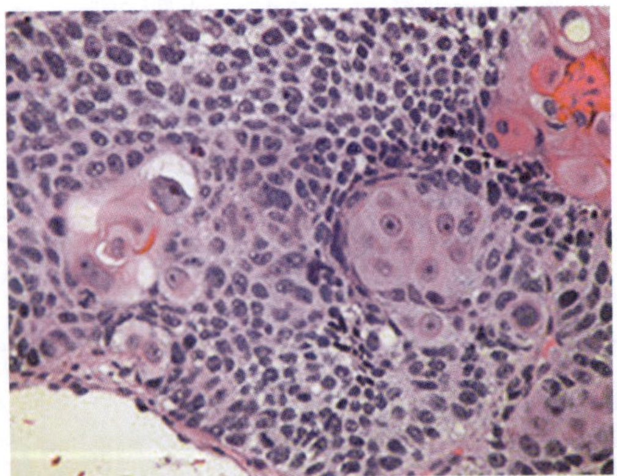

FIGURE 4.15 Microscopic picture of squamous cell carcinoma of lung

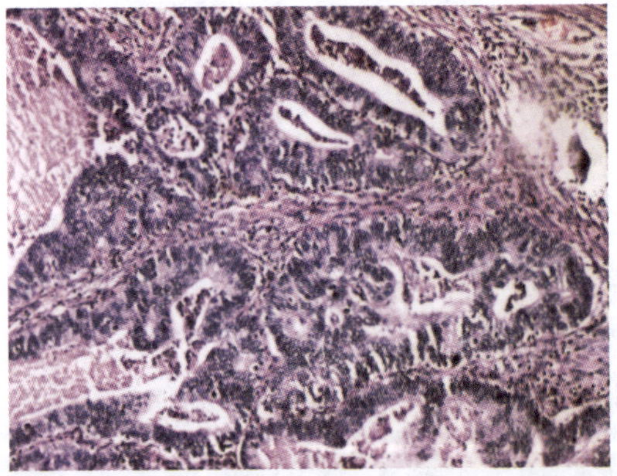

FIGURE 4.16 Microscopic picture of adenocarcinoma of lung

TABLE 4.1 Classification of pleural effusion

Condition	*Type of fluid*	*Associated conditions*
Inflammatory		
• Serofibrinous pleuritis	Serofibrinous exudate	Inflammation in adjacent lung
• Suppurative pleuritis (Empyema)	Pus	Suppurative infection in adjacent lung
• Hemorrhagic pleuritis	Bloody exudate	Tumor
Noninflammatory		
• Hydrothorax	Transudate	Congestive heart failure
• Hemothorax	Blood	Trauma
• Chylothorax	Lymph (chyle)	Tumor obstructed lymphatics

- Decreased lymphatic drainage as in carcinoma.

EMPYEMA

Empyema refers to purulent pleural exudates. This usually results from bacterial or fungal seeding of the pleural space. Most commonly it occurs by direct spread of infection from the parenchymal lung infections. Occasionally it can occur due to hematogenous spread. It is characterized by loculated yellow-green creamy pus. Microscopically it is characterized by sheets of neutrophils and other inflammatory cells. Culture of the pus will yield the causative organism. Empyema may resolve with antibiotics but may leave behind adhesions that will obliterate the pleural cavity.

CHAPTER 5

Cardiovascular System

ANATOMY

The human heart is a type of pump, which ejects blood through the body to maintain optimum circulation. It is divided into four chambers-right and left atria and ventricles. There are interatrial and interventricular septae dividing them. Tricuspid valve is present between right atrium and ventricle whereas mitral valve is seen between left atrium and ventricle. The semilunar valves, pulmonary valve and the aortic valves are present at the origin of the pulmonary artery and aorta from the right and left ventricles respectively. Normal heart weighs 250–300 g in females and 300–350 g in males. The thickness of the right ventricular wall is 0.3–0.5 cm and that of the left ventricle is 1.3–1.5 cm. Increase in the cardiac weight or size is called 'cardiomegaly'. Increased thickness of the ventricle or increased weight indicates hypertrophy and enlarged size of the heart chambers is called dilatation.

Conduction System

The sinoatrial pacemaker (SA node) is located at the junction of the right atrial appendage and superior vena cava. The atrioventricular (AV node) is located in the right atrium along the atrial septum. The bundle of His courses from the right atrium and divides into right and left bundle branches which arborize in the respective ventricles (Fig. 5.1).

Histology

The wall of the heart in all chambers consists of three main layers:

1. The endocardium
2. The intermediate muscular portion—the myocardium
3. The external portion—the pericardium.

Pericardium is divided into outer parietal and inner visceral pericardium and is lined by mesothelial cells.

The myocardium is made up of a collection of specialized muscle cells called cardiac myocytes. Intercalated disks join the adjacent cells. The endocardium is lined by the endothelial cells.

Blood Supply

The heart is supplied by right and left coronary arteries which are direct branches of aorta. The left main coronary artery further divides into left anterior descending (LAD) and left circumflex (LCX) arteries and supplies large part of the heart. The right coronary artery supplies right atrium and posterior third of the interventricular septum. Coronary veins run parallel to the arteries and drain into coronary sinus.

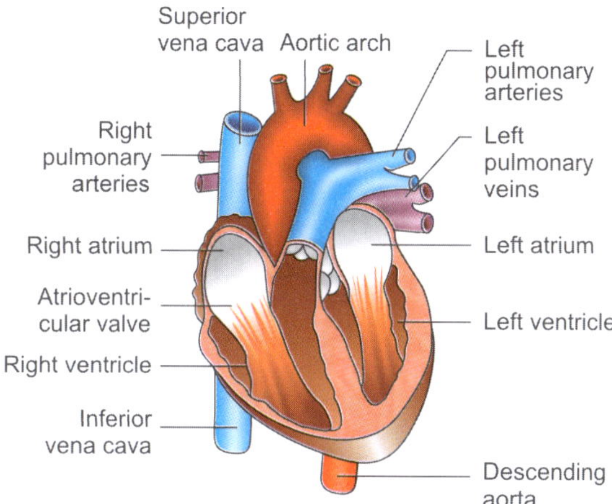

FIGURE 5.1 Diagrammatic representation of heart

PERICARDIAL DISEASE

Between the two mesothelial layers of the parietal and visceral pericardium is a potential space containing 30–50 mL of clear, straw-colored fluid. The pericardium helps in lubricating the surface of the heart and prevents deformation and dislocation of the heart and also acts as a barrier to the spread of infection.

Pericardial disease can present as:
- Acute pericarditis
- Pericardial effusion and cardiac tamponade
- Constrictive pericarditis.

Pericarditis is the inflammation of the pericardium. The major causes are:
- Infectious agents—viruses, pyogenic bacteria, tuberculosis, fungi and other parasites
- Immunologically mediated—rheumatic fever, scleroderma, systemic lupus erythematosus
- Metabolic—uremia, hypothyroidism
- Neoplasia—bronchogenic carcinoma
- Miscellaneous—myocardial infarction, trauma, following cardiac surgery, etc. (Table 5.1).

A pericardial effusion is a collection of fluid within the potential space of the serous pericardial sac. It commonly accompanies an episode of acute pericarditis. When a large volume collects rapidly in this space, ventricular filling is compromised leading to a condition known as cardiac tamponade.

Investigations

- ECG reveals low-voltage QRS complexes.
- *Chest X-ray*: shows large globular or pear-shaped heart with sharp outlines. Typically, the pulmonary veins are not distended.
- Echocardiography is the most useful technique for demonstrating the effusion and looking for evidence of tamponade.
- MRI should be considered if hemopericardium (blood in the pericardial space) or loculated pericardial effusions are suspected.
- Pericardiocentesis is the removal of pericardial fluid with aseptic technique under echocardiographic guidance. It is indicated when a tuberculous, malignant or purulent effusion is suspected.
- Pericardial biopsy may be needed if tuberculosis is suspected and pericardiocentesis not diagnostic.

Other tests include looking for underlying causes, e.g. blood cultures, autoantibody screen.

TABLE 5.1 Types of pericarditis

Type	*Type of collection*	*Causes*	*Morphology*
Serous	Collection of serous fluid	Immune mediated postviral	Neutrophils, lymphocytes and macrophages in the epicardial and pericardial surfaces
Serofibrinous/ fibrinous	Serous fluid mixed with fluid—yellow and cloudy	Post-MI, rheumatic fever, SLE	Surface is dry with fine granular roughening. Leukocytes, erythrocytes with fibrin can be seen
Purulent/ suppurative	Pus-like material	Suppurative inflammation	Serous surfaces—reddened, granular roughening. Leukocytes, erythrocytes with fibrin can be seen
Hemorrhagic	Hemorrhagic fluid material	Tumors, tuberculosis and bleeding diathesis	Blood mixed with a fibrinous or suppurative effusion. Cytology may yield neoplastic cells
Chronic adhesive	Fibrosis and organization with dense adhesions	Tuberculosis, suppuration	Pericardial fibrosis with obliteration of pericardial sac
Chronic constrictive	Dense fibrocalcific thickening	Tuberculosis and suppuration	Dense, adherent layer of scar with or without calcification (concretio cordis)

RHEUMATIC FEVER AND RHEUMATIC HEART DISEASE

Rheumatic fever (RF) is an acute, immunologically mediated, multisystem inflammatory disease that occurs a few weeks following an episode of group A streptococcal pharyngitis. It causes nonsuppurative inflammatory disease that affects the joints, tendons, arteries, connective tissue, heart, lungs, brain and serous membranes as sequelae to infection with group A beta hemolytic streptococci.

The important consequence of RF is chronic valvular deformities which produces permanent dysfunction. Despite its declining importance in industrialized countries, RF is a leading cause of death of heart disease in developing and underdeveloped countries due to poverty and overcrowding.

Rheumatic fever is diagnosed by a constellation of findings that includes major and minor criteria, so called Jones criteria (Table 5.2).

TABLE 5.2 Jones criteria

Major criteria	*Minor criteria*
Migratory polyarthritis	Arthralgia, fever
Carditis	Increased ESR and CRP
Erythema marginatum	Increased ASO titer
Subcutaneous nodules	Prolonged PR interval in ECG
Sydenham's chorea	Previous history of RF + throat culture for streptococci

Pathogenesis

It is suspected that acute rheumatic fever is a hypersensitivity reaction induced by group A streptococci. It is believed that antibodies directed against the M proteins of certain strains of streptococci cross react with glycoprotein antigens in the heart, joints and other tissues. So this supports the concept that RF results from an immune response against the streptococci.

Pathology

The inflammation is seen involving all the three layers of the heart, hence called pancarditis.

- *Rheumatic pericarditis*: In pericardium, the inflammation is accompanied by fibrinous or serofibrinous pericardial exudates, described as bread and butter pericarditis.

- *Rheumatic myocarditis*: Scattered Aschoff bodies which are pathognomonic of RF are seen in the interstitial connective tissue, often surrounding the blood vessels.

Aschoff bodies (Fig. 5.2A): They are spheroidal or fusiform distinct microscopic structures representing focal inflammatory lesions. They consist of foci of swollen eosinophilic collagen surrounded by lymphocytes, plasma cells and macrophages called Anitschkow cells (Fig. 5.2B).

Anitschkow cells have abundant cytoplasm and a central round to ovoid nucleus in which chromatin is seen in the form of a slender, wavy ribbon (hence called "caterpillar cells"). In cross-section, the chromatin appears as a small rounded body in the center of the nucleus looking like an 'owl's eye' (Fig. 5.3).

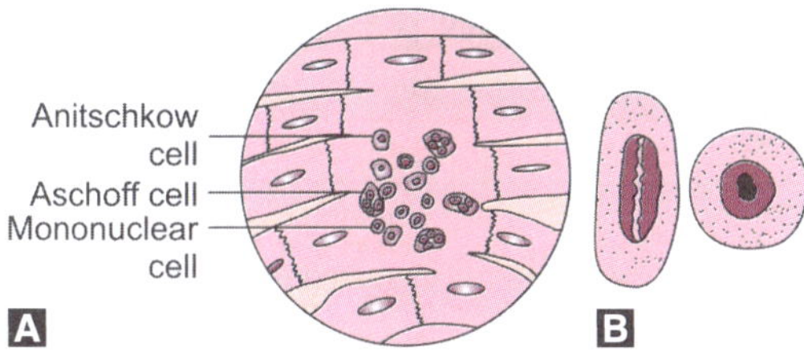

FIGURES 5.2A AND B Diagrammatic representation of (A) Aschoff body; and (B) Anitschkow cell. Note the caterpillar like chromatin in the Anitschkow cell in the longitudinal section

Evolution of a fully developed Aschoff body involves three stages all of which may be seen in the same heart at different stages. They are early exudative phase, intermediate proliferative phase and late fibrous stage.

- *Rheumatic endocarditis*: Involvement of endocardium and left sided valves results in fibrinoid necrosis with in the cusps on which are seen 1–2 mm vegetations along the line of closure (Fig. 5.4). Vegetations or verrucae are nothing but irregular, warty projections arising from precipitation of fibrin. Subendocardial lesions induce irregular thickenings in the left atrium called MacCallum plaques.

CHRONIC RHEUMATIC HEART DISEASE

Because of the organization of acute inflammation and fibrosis, the anatomical changes in the mitral or tricuspid valve are leaflet thickening, commissural fusion and thickening, shortening and fusion of chordae tendinae. In chronic rheumatic heart disease (RHD), the Aschoff bodies are replaced by fibrous scar.

Fibrous bridging and calcification across the commissures of the valves causes what is called "fish mouth" or "button hole" stenoses. This is most commonly seen in the left sided

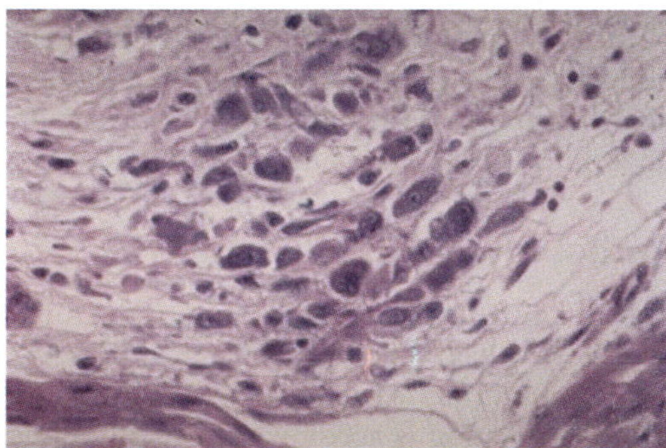

FIGURE 5.3 Microscopic picture of Aschoff body

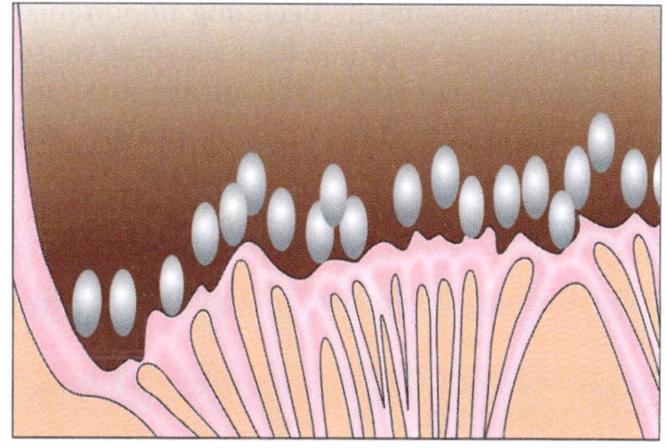

FIGURE 5.4 Vegetations are seen along the line of closure

valves, mitral and aortic and is rare in tricuspid and pulmonic valves.

Other clinical features seen in RF:

- Arthritis—migratory, no residual deformity' seen in large joints
- Erythema marginatum—erythematous skin lesions with raised margins
- Sydenham's chorea—fine purposeless involuntary movements
- Subcutaneous nodules—seen near elbow, painless.

The diagnosis is made by the evidence of a preceding group A streptococcal infection, with the presence of two of the major criteria or one major and two minor criteria.

Acute RF is most often seen in children between ages 5 and 15 years. The antibodies to streptococcal enzymes, such as streptolysin O and DNAse B are detected in the sera of most patients.

Acute carditis can manifest as pericardial friction rubs, weak heart sounds, tachycardia and arrhythmias. Myocarditis can cause cardiac dilatation that may lead to heart failure. Patients from chronic carditis suffer from arrhythmias, thromboembolic complications and infective endocarditis.

Treatment

Surgical repair of diseased valves by incising the fused mitral valve commissures and replacement with prosthetic devices.

INFECTIVE ENDOCARDITIS

Definition

Infective endocarditis (IE) is characterized by invasion or colonization of heart valves or endocardium by an infective organism.

Classification

It is classified on clinical grounds into acute and subacute IE (Table 5.3).

TABLE 5.3 Acute and subacute infective endocarditis

Acute	*Subacute*
Highly virulent organism	Arthralgia, fever
Previously normal heart	Previously diseased heart
Destructive and fulminant	Less fulminant
Death within days—weeks in more than 50%	Protracted course, may recover with appropriate antibiotic therapy

Predisposing Factors

1. Underlying heart disorders—rheumatic heart disease, artificial valves, bicuspid aortic valve, myxomatous mitral valve, degenerative calcific valvular stenosis and others.
2. Intravenous drug abuse.
3. Host factors such as immunodeficiency, malignancy, diabetes mellitus, neutropenia.
4. Bacteremia and septicemia—severe pneumonia, dental sepsis, lung abscess and others.

Causative Organisms

- *Streptococcus viridans*: Infects previously damaged or abnormal valves.
- *Staphylococcus aureus*: May infect damaged or healthy valves. Most commonly causes endocarditis in intravenous drug abusers.
- HACEK group (*Haemophilus, Actinobacillus, Cardiobacterium, Eikenella* and *Kingella*), enterococci.
- Coagulase negative staphylococci, e.g. *S. epidermidis*—infects most commonly the artificial valves.
- Gram negative bacilli and fungi.
- *Culture negative endocarditis*: In around 10 percent of the cases, no organism is identified.

Pathology

The disease is characterized by friable, bulky and destructive vegetations on the valve cusps

that can extend onto the chordae tendinae. These vegetations consist of microorganisms, fibrin, platelet, inflammatory cells and they cause destruction of the leaflets producing valvular dysfunction. Vegetations may be single or multiple and may involve more than one valve. Fungal endocarditis causes larger vegetations. The aortic and mitral valves are the most common sites of infection. The right sided heart valves are involved in intravenous drug abusers (Fig. 5.5).

Complications

1. *Ring abscess*: Vegetations erode into the myocardium below to cause an abscess.
2. Perforation of valve cusps and valve dehiscence.
3. *Systemic emboli*: Because of the friability of the vegetations they can form emboli and cause infarction in the brain, kidneys and other tissues.
4. *Septic infarcts*: At the site of infarcts, abscesses may develop.
5. Suppurative pericarditis.
6. *Glomerulonephritis*: Immune mediated.

Clinical Features

1. Fever, fatigue, weight loss, flu like syndrome, change of heart murmurs.
2. *Clinical findings secondary to microemboli*: Petechiae, splinter hemorrhages (red, linear or flame shaped streaks in the nail bed of digits), Osler nodes (subcutaneous nodules in the pulp of the digits), Janeway lesions (hemorrhagic nontender lesions on the palms or soles), Roth spots (retinal hemorrhages).

Laboratory Investigations

Blood culture helps to identify the causative organism. A positive blood culture in three consecutive samples is diagnostic.

The diagnosis is established based on Duke's criteria which have major and minor signs.

Prevention

Prophylactic antibiotics in patients having artificial valves or any cardiac anomaly who is about to undergo some surgical, dental or other invasive procedures.

ARTERIOSCLEROSIS

Arteriosclerosis indicates thickening of the arteries and loss of elasticity. Three patterns have been recognized:

1. Atherosclerosis
2. *Arteriolosclerosis*: Usually associated with hypertension
3. *Monckeberg medial calcific sclerosis*: Typically occurs in old age. There is calcification in the media of small to medium sized arteries. It is clinically insignificant (Fig. 5.6).

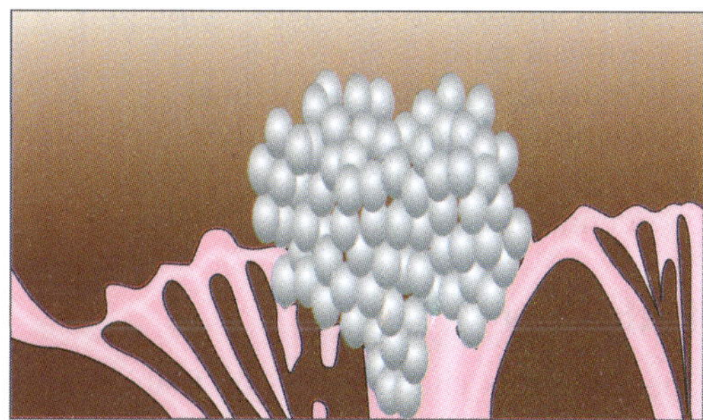

FIGURE 5.5 Vegetations in infective endocarditis

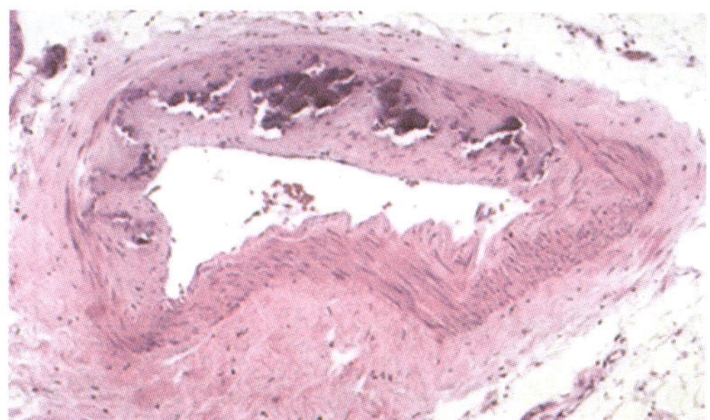

FIGURE 5.6 Microscopy of Monckeberg medial calcific sclerosis

Atherosclerosis

Atherosclerosis is a slowly progressive disease characterized by lesions in the intima of the large to medium sized muscular and large elastic arteries. These lesions are called atheromas or atheromatous plaques or fibrofatty plaques. These plaques protrude into the vascular lumens, obstruct them and also weaken the underlying media. It involves arteries such as abdominal aorta, coronary arteries, descending thoracic aorta, popliteal arteries, internal carotid arteries and so on.

Major consequences of atherosclerosis are:
1. Myocardial infarction
2. Cerebrovascular accidents
3. Peripheral vascular occlusive disorders
4. Aneurysms.

Risk Factors

They can be divided into major nonmodifiable factors, potentially controllable factors and modifiable factors (Table 5.4).

Pathogenesis

There are many theories and hypothesis. The most widely accepted hypothesis is response to injury hypothesis: chronic inflammatory response of the arterial wall to some form of EC injury. The sequential events are as follows.

- Focal endothelial injury causes endothelial dysfunction, increasing endothelial permeability and expression of leukocyte adhesion molecules.
- Blood monocytes and other leukocytes adhere to the altered endothelial cells.
- Monocytes migrate into the intima and transform to macrophages, engulf lipid to form foam cells.
- Lipoproteins insudate into vessel walls at the foci of injury.
- Macrophages oxidize the lipoproteins.
- Platelets get adhered to the areas of endothelial injury.
- Activated platelets and macrophages release factors such as platelet-derived growth factor (PDGF) that cause medial smooth muscle cells (SMCs) to migrate into the intima.
- SMCs proliferate in the intima and elaborate extracellular matrix (ECM).
- Lipids accumulate with in the cells (SMCs and macrophages) and also extracellularly.

TABLE 5.4 Risk factors of atherosclerosis

Nonmodifiable	*Potentially modifiable*	*Modifiable*
Old age	Diabetes mellitus	Physical activity
Gender	Hypertension	Stress
Family history	Smoking	Carbohydrate intake
Genetic causes	Hyperlipidemia	Unsaturated fat intake
Homocystinemia	Obesity	Alcohol

Morphology

An atheroma consists of a raised focal lesion initiating with in the intima, having a soft, yellow, core of lipid (cholesterol and cholesterol esters), covered by a firm, white fibrous cap. The size of these varies from 0.3 to 1.5 cm in diameter but sometimes coalesce to become larger masses.

- Fatty streak is the earliest lesion characterized by multiple thin yellow spots with in the intima.
- Complicated plaque indicates advanced lesion. The changes include fibrosis of the plaque, calcification, ulceration, formation of thrombus, hemorrhage with in the plaque, thinning of the media and formation of aneurysms.

Atheromas have three main components:
1. Cells—macrophages, smooth muscle cells, other leukocytes.
2. Extracellular matrix (ECM)—collagen, elastic fibers and proteoglycans.
3. Intracellular and extracellular lipid.

Atheromatous plaques have superficial fibrous caps containing SMCs, leukocytes and

dense connective tissue overlying necrotic cores, containing dead cells, lipid, cholesterol clefts, lipid-laden foam cells and plasma proteins. Proliferation of small blood vessels can be seen at the intimal-medial interface (Figs 5.7A and B).

Clinical Features

Atherosclerosis can begin in childhood but is typically asymptomatic for many decades. It can manifest as:

- Insidious narrowing of vascular lumens, e.g. gangrene of lower leg due to narrowing of popliteal arteries.
- Sudden occlusion of vascular lumens due to plaque rupture or erosion followed by superimposed thrombus, e.g. myocardial infarction after a disrupted coronary atheroma.
- Aneurysm formation and their possible rupture due to weakening of the vessels, e.g. abdominal aortic aneurysm.
- Source of thromboemboli to some distal organ causing damage, e.g. mesenteric occlusion causing bowel infarction and renal ischemia due to renal artery occlusion.

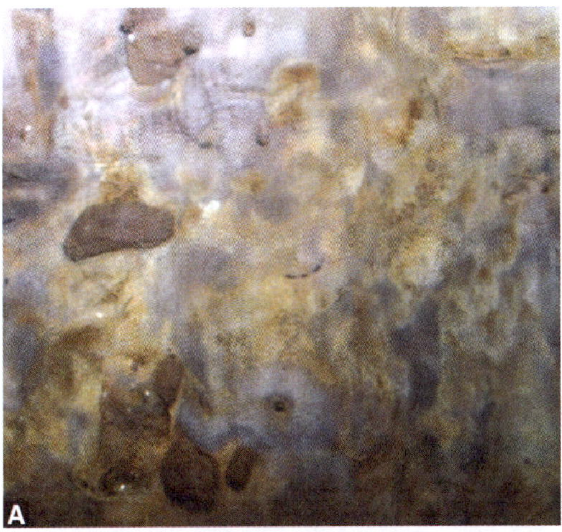

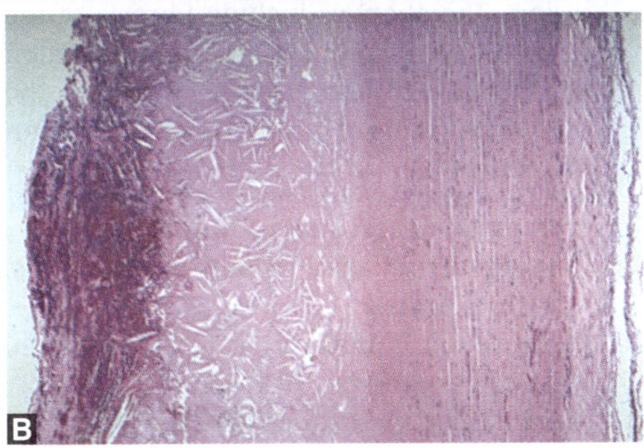

FIGURES 5.7A AND B Gross photograph of atheroma aorta

ISCHEMIC HEART DISEASE

It is the term used for a group of related syndromes resulting from myocardial ischemia. There is an imbalance between the supply and demand of the heart for oxygenated blood. In ischemia, the tissue not only subjected to insufficient oxygen but also insufficient nutrients and inadequate removal of metabolites.

Causes

The most common cause is coronary artery atherosclerosis (90%). The less common causes include coronary vasospasm, coronary thromboembolism and cyanotic heart diseases.

The common conditions under this disease are:

1. Myocardial infarction
2. Angina pectoris
3. Chronic IHD with heart failure
4. Sudden cardiac death.

Pathogenesis

The pathogenetic mechanisms include interaction between fixed epicardial coronary narrowing, thrombosis overlying a disrupted atherosclerotic plaque, platelet aggregation and vasospasm.

- *Fixed coronary narrowing*: When the obstruction is 75 percent or more, it causes ischemia induced by exercise. A 90 percent obstruction can lead to ischemia even at rest. It is seen most commonly in left anterior descending artery, left circumflex and right coronary artery. A single artery, two arteries or all three may get involved.

- *Disrupted atherosclerotic plaque*: Disruption may be in the form of rupture of the plaque, erosion, ulceration and hemorrhage into the atheroma. This leads to thrombogenesis and thrombi is formed over the disrupted atherosclerotic plaque. This converts partial obstruction into a complete one.
- *Platelet aggregation and vasospasm*: They play a minor role in causing coronary obstruction.

Angina Pectoris

Angina pectoris is a symptom complex characterized by pain (constricting, squeezing or choking type) that typically occurs in the substernal portion of the chest and may radiate to the left arm, jaw, and epigastrium. It is the most common symptom of ischemic heart disease. A patient with typical angina pectoris exhibits recurrent episodes of chest pain, usually brought on by increased physical activity or emotional excitement. The pain is of limited duration (1 to 15 minutes). It is caused by transient myocardial ischemia which falls short of causing necrosis (infarction).

There are three types of angina pectoris:

1. *Stable angina*: Most common form and caused by chronic coronary stenosis due to atherosclerosis. The patient experiences pain during physical activity and emotional excitement and is relieved by rest or nitroglycerin (potent vasodilator).
2. *Prinzmetal's variant angina*: Uncommon pattern occurring at rest and is due to coronary vasospasm. It is not related to physical activity and is relieved by nitroglycerin and calcium channel blockers.
3. *Unstable or crescendo angina*: It occurs at rest and of prolonged duration. It is caused by sudden change in the plaque morphology which severely reduces coronary blood flow. It is often a prodrome of acute MI and is, therefore, sometimes called preinfarction angina.

Sudden Cardiac Death

It involves a coronary lesion in which disrupted plaque with thrombus and possibly embolus has caused regional myocardial ischemia. It induces a fatal ventricular arrhythmia.

Myocardial Infarction

Myocardial infarction (MI) is the death of cardiac muscle resulting from ischemia.

There are two patterns of myocardial infarction. They are:

1. Transmural.
2. Subendocardial.

Transmural infarction involves the full thickness of the ventricular wall in the distribution of a single coronary artery. It is usually associated with acute change in plaque morphology and formation of thrombus over a disrupted atherosclerotic plaque.

Subendocardial infarction involves inner one-third or at most half of the ventricular wall. It may extend beyond the territory of a single coronary artery.

Age Incidence

Myocardial infarction can occur at any age but frequency increases with age.

Predisposing Factors

The predisposing factors of MI are, cigarette smoking, hypertension, diabetes mellitus, hypercholesterolemia, hyperlipoproteinemia and others.

Women are usually protected in their reproductive years. Following menopause, due to decrease in estrogen, there can be raised development of coronary artery disease.

Pathogenesis

It has already been discussed under atherosclerosis (Fig. 5.8).

Myocardial Response

Myocardium undergoes various biochemical, morphological and functional alterations in response to ischemia.

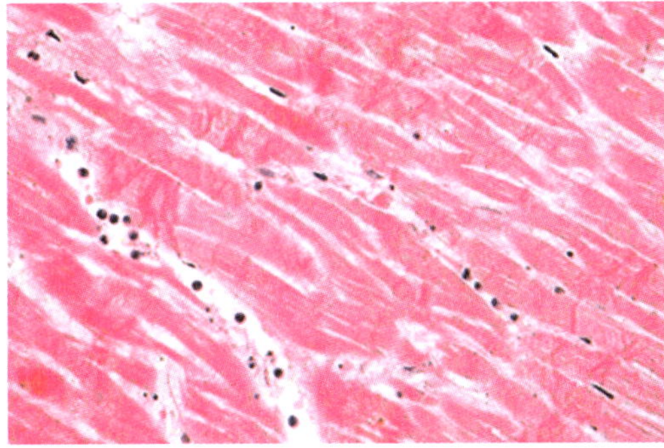

FIGURE 5.8 Microscopy of myocardial infarction

- *Biochemical changes*: The early biochemical consequence is the cessation of aerobic glycolysis leading to inadequate ATP (adenosine triphosphate) and accumulation of breakdown products like lactic acid.
- Morphological changes (Table 5.5).
- *Functional changes*: There is loss of contractility within 60 seconds. Severe ischemia lasting for 20–40 minutes leads to cell death.

Clinical Features

Patients have sudden precordial or retrosternal chest pain which radiates to the left shoulder, left arm, jaw, epigastrium and back with sweating and difficulty in breathing. Pulse is weak, rapid and thready. In conditions like diabetes mellitus and old age, the patients may

TABLE 5.5 Morphological changes in MI

Duration	*Gross features*	*Light microscopy*	*Electron microscopy*
Reversible injury 0–30 min	None	None	Mitochondrial Swell relaxed myofibrils, glycogen loss
Irreversible injury 30 min to 4 hours	None	Variable	Disruption of sarcolemma, waviness of fibers at border Mitochondrial amorphous densities
4–12 hours	Occasional dark-mottled area	Onset of coagulation necrosis, edema and hemorrhage	
12–24 hours	Dark-mottled area	Coagulation necrosis with pyknosis of nuclei and myocyte hypereosinophilia and contraction band necrosis	
24–92 hours	Dark-mottled area with central yellow areas	Coagulation necrosis with loss of nuclei and striations and neutrophilic infiltrate	
3–7 days	Hyperemic border separates infracted area	Disintegration of dead fibers, dying neutrophils, phagocytosis of dead cells by macrophages	
7–10 days	Central yellow areas with red margins	Early formation of granulation tissue	
10–14 days	Red-gray infarct border	Granulation tissue	
2–8 weeks	Gray-white scar	Deposition of collagen	
> 2 months	Complete scarring	Dense collagenous scar	

TABLE 5.6 Characteristics of biomarkers

Characterisitic	CK	CK-2	LDH, LDH-2	Myoglobin	Troponin
Molecular weight	86,000	86,000	3,35,000	18,000	23,000(I) 42,000(T)
Hours until peak concentration	10–24	10–24	72–144	6–9	24–48
Days until return to reference limit	3–4	2–3	8–12	7–10	

be asymptomatic and this is called silent myocardial infarction.

ECG changes: Elevation or depression of ST segment, T wave inversion and appearance of new Q waves are some of the common findings.

Laboratory tests: It is based on measuring the blood levels of enzymes which get released into the circulation from the injured myocardial cells through the damaged membranes. These are called biomarkers. The common biomarkers that are seen elevated are (Table 5.6):

1. Creatinine kinase (CK - BB/1, CK - MB/2, CK - MM/3)
   CK - MB or CK - 2 is most useful.
2. Lactate dehydrogenase
3. Troponin T and troponin I
4. Myoglobin
5. Myosin light chain
6. Aspartate aminotransferase.

Complications of Myocardial Infarction

1. Cardiac arrhythmias
2. Myocardial rupture
3. Contractile dysfunction
4. Pericarditis
5. Infarct expansion
6. Ventricular aneurysm
7. Progressive late heart failure
8. Mural thrombus.

ANEURYSMS

Definition

Aneurysms are defined as localized abnormal permanent dilatation of blood vessels or the wall of the heart.

TABLE 5.7 Classification of aneurysms

Criteria	*Examples*
Nature of the wall	• True aneurysm (bounded by arterial wall components or attenuated wall of the heart), e.g. atherosclerotic, syphilitic and congenital. • False aneurysm (bounded by fibrous tissue), e.g. post-MI rupture
Morphology	• Berry aneurysm—spherical (1–10 mm) • Saccular (5–20 cm)—spherical • Fusiform (up to 20 cm)—spindle shaped • Cirsoid – irregular • Cylindrical
Etiology	• Atherosclerosis • Syphilis • Trauma • Congenital • Infective (mycotic aneurysm) • Aortic dissection • Vasculitides

Classification

Based on the components of their lining, macroscopic shape or size and the etiology they are classified as follows (Table 5.7 and Fig. 5.9).

Abdominal Aortic Aneurysms

Atherosclerosis is the most frequent etiology of aneurysms and atherosclerotic aneurysms occur most frequently in abdominal aorta.

Site

It is usually positioned below the renal arteries and above the bifurcation of aorta.

Morphology

They are saccular or fusiform and up to 15 cm in diameter.

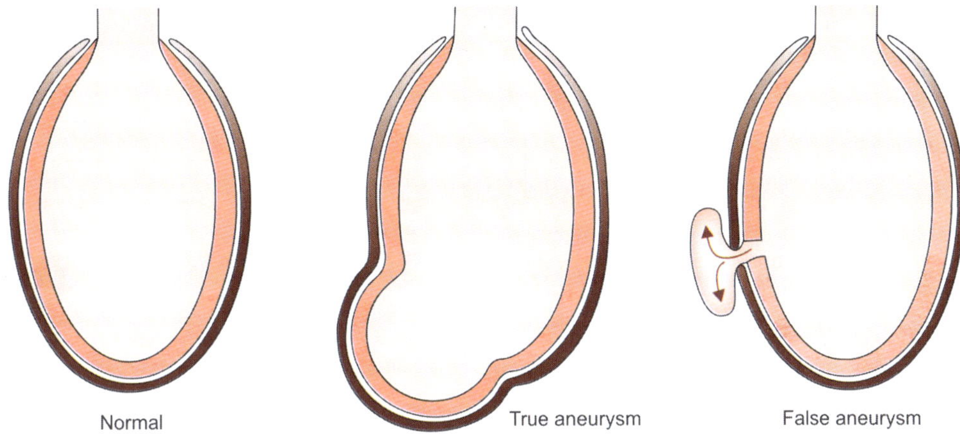

FIGURE 5.9 Diagrammatic representation of true and false aneurysms

Pathogenesis

Weakening of tunica media by atherosclerotic lesions.

Clinical Features

Rupture with massive hemorrhage, pressure effect on adjacent structures like ureter, obstruction of vessels like iliac, renal, mesenteric leading to ischemia, thrombosis and embolism.

Syphilitic (Luetic) Aneurysms

It is seen in tertiary stage of syphilis.

Site

It is confined to thoracic aorta.

Morphology

It can be saccular or fusiform.

Pathogenesis

Syphilitic involvement of vasa vasorum in the adventitia of aorta induces obliterative endarteritis. The lumen gets narrowed and aortic media suffers ischemic injury with loss of medial elastic fibers and muscle cells followed by inflammation and scarring. Once the media gets destroyed, the aorta losses its elasticity, becomes dilated causing syphilitic aneurysm. The contraction of these fibrous scars leads to wrinkling of the intervening segments of aortic intima and appears as a tree bark grossly.

These aneurysms are usually accompanied by aortic valve ring dilatation with massive left ventricular hypertrophy, referred to as "Cor bovinum" (cow's heart).

Clinical Features

Encroachment on mediastinal structures, erosion of bones like ribs and vertebral bodies, rupture.

Aortic Dissection (Dissecting Hematoma)

Aortic dissection is characterized by formation of a blood filled channel with in the aortic wall between the laminar planes of tunica media, which often rupture causing massive hemorrhage.

Pathogenesis

Hypertension is the major risk factor. In Marfan syndrome, an autosomal dominant disease,

the most frequent pre-existing lesion is cystic medial degeneration characterized by elastic tissue fragmentation.

Morphology

An intimal tear is the initial event. These tears are transverse or oblique with sharp, jagged edges. The dissecting hematoma spreads between the middle and outer thirds of the laminar planes of aorta. Sometimes the blood reruptures into the lumen due to a second intimal tear to produce a "double barreled aorta".

Classification (Fig. 5.10)

1. Type A
2. Type B

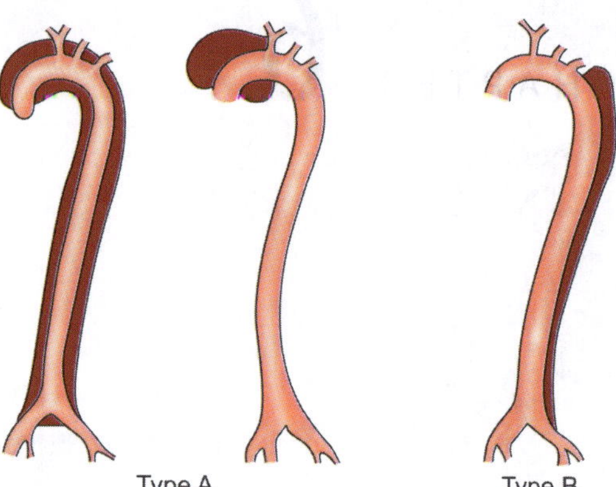

FIGURE 5.10 Diagrammatic representation of types of dissecting aneurysm

Clinical Features

The classical clinical symptom is sudden excruciating pain in the anterior chest, radiating to the back. The common cause of death is rupture of the dissection outward into any of the three body cavities (pleural, peritoneal or pericardial).

CHAPTER 6

Gastrointestinal Tract

NORMAL ANATOMY

The gastrointestinal tract consists of the mouth, esophagus, stomach, small intestine, large intestine, appendix, rectum and anus (Fig. 6.1).

HISTOLOGY

Histologically, the entire gastrointestinal tract (GIT) consists of four layers, namely mucosa, submucosa, muscularis and serosa.

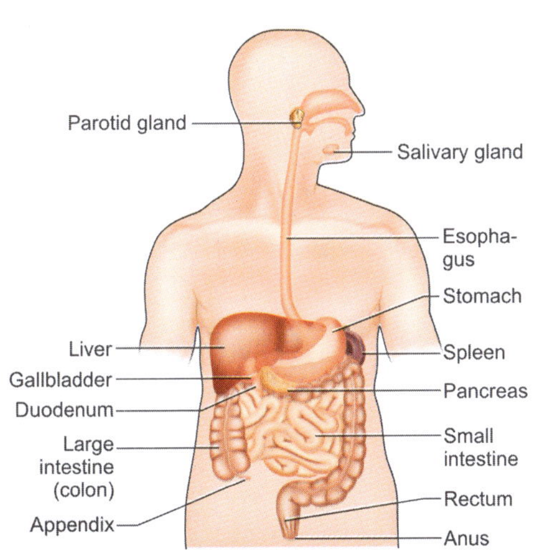

FIGURE 6.1 Anatomy of gastrointestinal system

Blood Supply

The GIT is supplied mainly by the celiac trunk, superior and inferior mesenteric arteries. The venous blood is drained by the portal veins. The lymphatics drain mainly into the thoracic duct.

Nerve Supply

The innervation of the GIT is mainly derived by the autonomic nervous system.

Functions

The main function of the GIT is mastication in the mouth, digestion in the stomach, absorption in the small intestine and excretion by the large intestine, rectum and anus.

PATHOLOGY

Peptic Ulcer

An ulcer is defined as a discontinuity in the lining epithelium.

Peptic ulcers are chronic ulcers that occur in any part of the GIT exposed to the aggressive action of acid and peptic juices.

Sites of occurrence of peptic ulcer in the GIT are:

- First part of duodenum—Most common
- Antrum of the stomach
- At the gastroesophageal junction, in cases of Barret's esophagus (A condition, wherein there is metaplasia and replacement of squamous epithelium by columnar epithelium in the lower part of the esophagus).

ETIOLOGY AND PATHOGENESIS

Peptic ulcers are produced by an imbalance between the gastroduodenal mucosal defense mechanisms and the damaging forces, particularly gastric acid and pepsin.

- *Helicobacter pylori infection*: These bacteria are considered to be the most important cause of peptic ulcer. The mechanisms with which it produces the disease are:
  - *H. pylori* does not invade the mucosa, but it produces cytokines, such as interleukin-6 (IL-6) and tumor necrosis factor (TNF) which cause inflammation.
  - Several bacterial gene products are involved in causing epithelial cell injury and induction of inflammation.
  - *H. pylori* increase the gastric acid secretion and impairs the duodenal bicarbonate production. This favors further colonization by *H. pylori.*
- Chronic use of drugs, such as non-steroidal anti-inflammatory drugs (NSAIDs) act as direct irritants producing peptic ulcer.
- Cigarette smoking and alcohol also play an important role in the causation of peptic ulcer.
- Long time and high dosage use of corticosteroids.
- Chronic diseases such as alcoholic cirrhosis, chronic obstructive pulmonary disease and chronic renal failure are associated with peptic ulcer disease.
- Psychological stress.

Morphology

About 98 percent of the peptic ulcers are located in the first part of duodenum or in the stomach in the ratio of 4:1.

Duodenal ulcers are located most commonly in the anterior wall. Gastric ulcers are predominantly located on the lesser curvature.

Gross

A classical peptic ulcer is round to oval in shape with sharply punched out edges and a clean smooth base. The margins of the ulcer are in level with the surrounding mucosa.

Microscopy

In an active peptic ulcer with necrosis, 4 zones can be demonstrated:

- Presence of superficial necrotic fibrinoid debris in the base and the margins of the ulcer.
- Next is a zone of nonspecific inflammatory infiltrate, with predominantly neutrophils.
- Deeper layer of granulation tissue.
- Granulation tissue resting on a deeper layer of scar tissue formed due to fibrosis.

Clinical Features

Burning in the epigastric region or aching pain are the early features. Nausea, vomiting, belching, and weight loss can occur.

Complications are hemorrhage, perforation and anemia.

TYPHOID (ENTERIC FEVER)

Enteric fever is an acute infection caused by *Salmonella typhi* (typhoid fever) or *Salmonella paratyphi* (paratyphoid fever).

Etiopathogenesis

The route of entry of the organism is through ingestion of contaminated food or water. In the initial 2 weeks, the bacteria invade the lymphoid follicles and payer's patches of the small intestine. Later, the bacteria invade the bloodstream causing bacteremia resulting in typical 'step ladder' kind of fever in typhoid.

Morphology

The lesions caused by typhoid are seen mainly in the intestine; some cases also show lesions in other organs.

Gross

Terminal ileum is affected most commonly, though the jejunum and colon are rarely involved. The site of activity is the Payer's patches, which shows oval typhoid ulcers. Typically, these ulcers have their long axis along the length of their bowel. The base of the ulcer is black due to sloughed mucosa. The margins of the ulcer are slightly raised due to inflammatory edema. The regional lymph nodes are enlarged (Fig. 6.2).

Microscopy

Hyperemia, edema and cellular proliferation consisting of histiocytes, lymphocytes and plasma cells is seen. In the peripheral blood smear, typhoid fever typically causes reduction in neutrophil count (neutropenia).

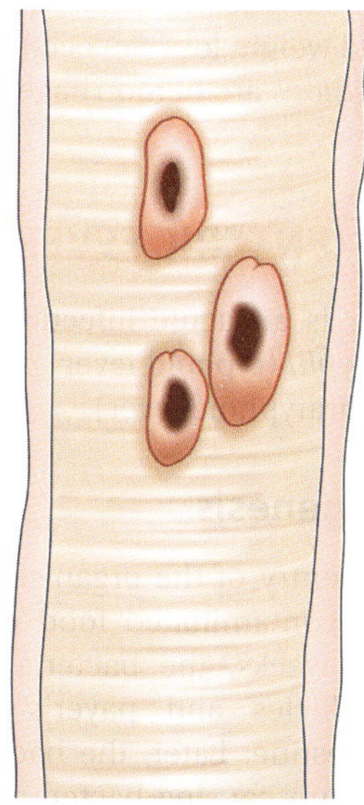

FIGURE 6.2 Diagrammatic representation of oval typhoid ulcer

Complications of Intestinal Lesions

- Perforation of ulcer.
- Hemorrhage.

Typhoid lesions in other organs include:
- Mesenteric lymph node—hemorrhagic lymphadenitis.
- Liver—foci of parenchymal necrosis.
- Gall bladder—typhoid cholecystitis.
- Spleen—splenomegaly with reactive hyperplasia.
- Bones—osteitis.

CARCINOMA ESOPHAGUS

Esophageal carcinomas constitute 6 percent of all gastrointestinal malignancies.

SQUAMOUS CELL CARCINOMA

Squamous cell carcinoma (SCC) is the most common malignant tumor in the esophagus. SCC is seen in adults, more than 50 years of age and more common in men than women.

Etiopathogenesis

Esophageal carcinoma can result from a number of factors and so it is said to be multifactorial.

Factors associated with the development of esophageal squamous cell carcinoma.

Dietary

- Deficiency of vitamins (A, C, riboflavin, thiamine, pyridoxine).
- Deficiency of trace elements (zinc and molybdenum).
- High content of nitrites, nitrosamines.
- Fungal contamination of food.
- Betel chewing.

Lifestyle

- Burning hot beverages or food.
- Alcohol consumption.
- Tobacco use.
- Urban environment.

Esophageal Disorders

- Long-standing esophagitis.
- Achalasia cardia.
- Plummer-Vinson syndrome.

Genetic Predisposition

Morphology: SCC begins as a gray-white plaque-like thickening of the esophageal mucosa. Lesions subsequently extend longitudinally and circumferentially and invade deeply.

Gross: It can be polypoidal in 60 percent of cases, ulcerative in 25 percent of cases or diffusely infiltrative in 15 percent of cases.

Microscopy: These tumors resemble SCC seen anywhere else, usually being moderately to well differentiated.

Clinical features: SCC is insidious in onset with symptoms of dysphagia, obstruction, weight loss, hemorrhage and sepsis.

ADENOCARCINOMA

Etiopathogenesis

Adenocarcinoma mainly occurs due to dysplastic changes in Barrett's esophagus.

Morphology

Gross

Adenocarcinoma can present in many ways, such as exophytic nodules, ulcerative or infiltrative.

Microscopy

Tumor cells are seen arranged in acinar pattern with mucin producing glands. Some cases can show signet ring cell differentiation.

Clinical Features

Adenocarcinoma of esophagus typically arises in patients above 40 years of age and is more common in women with symptoms similar to SCC.

CARCINOMA STOMACH

The gastric carcinoma constitutes 90–95 percent of gastric malignancies. The rest are lymphomas, carcinoids or gastrointestinal stromal tumors.

Etiopathogenesis

Risk factors for the development of gastric carcinoma.

Environmental Factors

- Infection by *H. pylori.*
- Diet
  - Nitrites in preserved food
  - Smoked and salted food, pickled vegetables, chilli, pepper
  - Lack of fresh fruits and vegetables.
- Low socioeconomic status.
- Cigarette smoking.

Host Factors

- Chronic gastritis
- Partial gastrectomy
- Gastric adenoma
- Barrett esophagus.

Genetic Factors

- Slightly increased risk with blood group A.
- Family history of gastric cancer.
- Familial gastric cancer syndrome.

Morphology

Gastric carcinoma is seen in the antrum and pylorus in 60 percent of the cases. Less commonly it is also seen involving the cardia or the body and the fundus of the stomach. Lesser curvature is involved in 40 percent of cases whereas greater curvature is involved in 12 percent of cases. Thus, the most favored location for the occurrence of gastric cancer is the lesser curvature of the antropyloric region.

Classification of Gastric Carcinoma

Based on the Depth of Invasion

- *Early gastric carcinoma:* Tumor is confined to the mucosa and submucosa.
- *Advanced gastric carcinoma:* Tumor extends beyond the submucosa into the muscularis and serosa.

Based on the Macroscopic Growth Pattern

- *Exophytic*: Tumor is large, protruding into the lumen.
- Depressed/flat.
- Excavated/ulcerative (Figs 6.3 and 6.4).

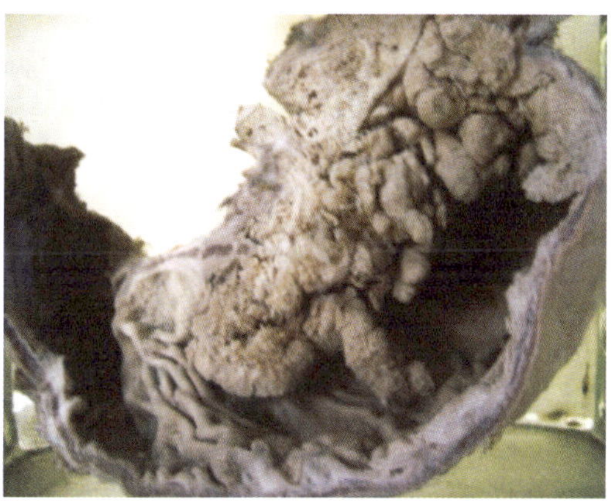

FIGURE 6.3 Gross picture of carcinoma stomach showing exophytic growth

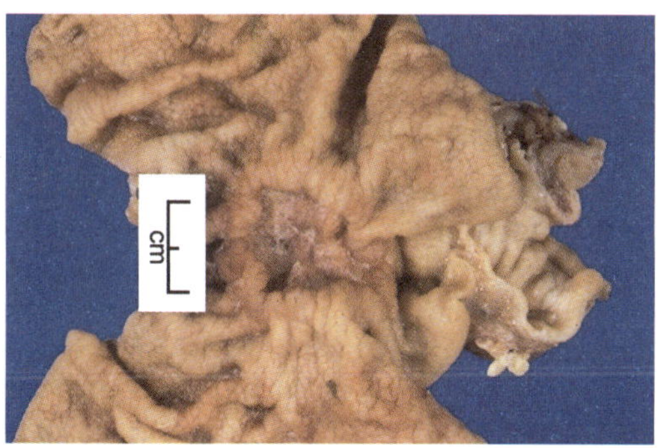

FIGURE 6.4 Gross picture of malignant ulcer in the stomach

Based on the Histologic Subtype

- *Intestinal type:* Tumor cells are mucin producing and gland forming. This microscopic type usually has an expansile type of growth and is preceded by intestinal metaplasia. This type has a mean age incidence of 55 years with male: female=2:1.
- *Diffuse type:* In this microscopic subtype, the tumor cells are poorly differentiated, single signet ring cells producing mucin. This type, usually, has an infiltrative growth pattern with a mean age incidence of 48 years and a male: female = 1:1 (Fig. 6.5).

Spread and metastasis: Irrespective of the classification, all gastric carcinomas eventually penetrate the muscularis to involve the serosa and then to the regional lymph nodes and later to the distant lymph nodes. Many a times, metastatizes to the left supraclavicular lymph node called *Virchow's node* and is the first clinical manifestation of the disease. The tumor can also metastatize to the periumbilical region to form subcutaneous nodules. This nodule is called *Sister Mary Joseph's nodule*, after the nun who noted this lesion as the metastatic marker. It can also involve the liver and the lungs. Metastasis to bilateral ovaries is called *Krukenberg tumor*.

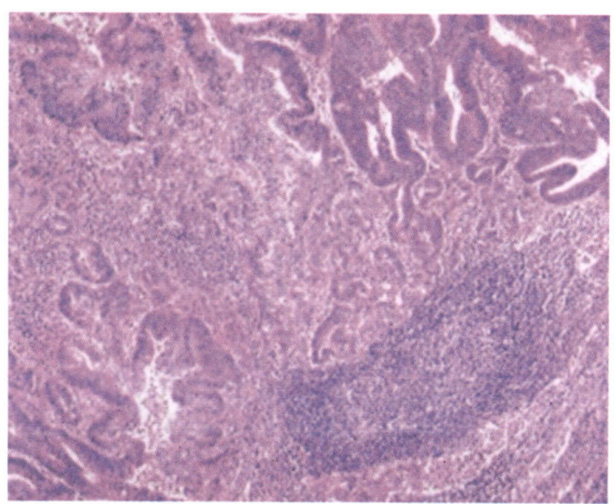

FIGURE 6.5 Microscopy of carcinoma stomach

Clinical Features

Carcinoma stomach is insidious in onset exhibiting weight loss, abdominal pain, anorexia, vomiting, altered bowel habits, dysphagia, anemia and hemorrhage.

Prognosis

Early gastric cancer has a 5 years survival rate of 90 to 95 percent. Advanced gastric cancer has a 5 years survival rate of less than 15 percent.

CARCINOMA COLON

Ninety-eight percent of all cancers in the GIT are adenocarcinomas.

Etiopathogenesis

The peak age incidence of carcinoma colon is between 60 and 79 years.

Factors predisposing to the development of colon cancer:

Dietary

- Excess dietary caloric intake relative to requirements.
- Low content of vegetable fiber.
- Corresponding high intake of refined carbohydrates.
- Intake of red meat.
- Reduced intake of protective micronutrients.

Epidemiological

Increased incidence is seen in Japanese as compared to inhabitants of the United States.

Morphology: The distribution of cancer in colorectum is as follows:

- Cecum/ascending colon—22 percent
- Transverse colon—11 percent
- Desscending colon—6 percent
- Rectsigmoid—55 percent
- Others—6 percent.

Gross: Tumors in the right side of the colon (proximal part) grow as polypoid, exophytic masses that extend along the capacious cecum and ascending colon. In this type, obstruction is rare (Fig. 6.6.).

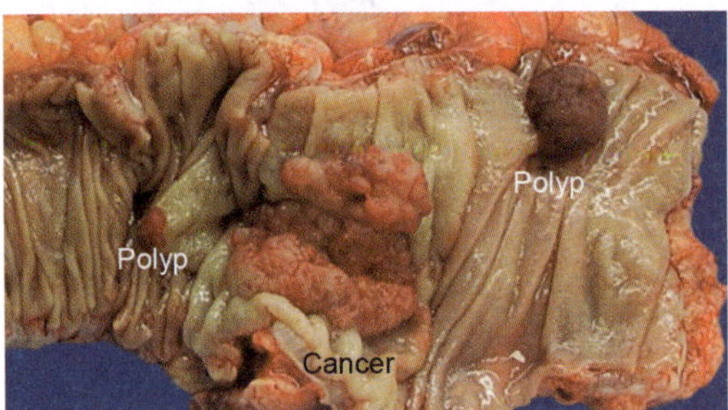

FIGURE 6.6 Gross picture of carcinoma colon

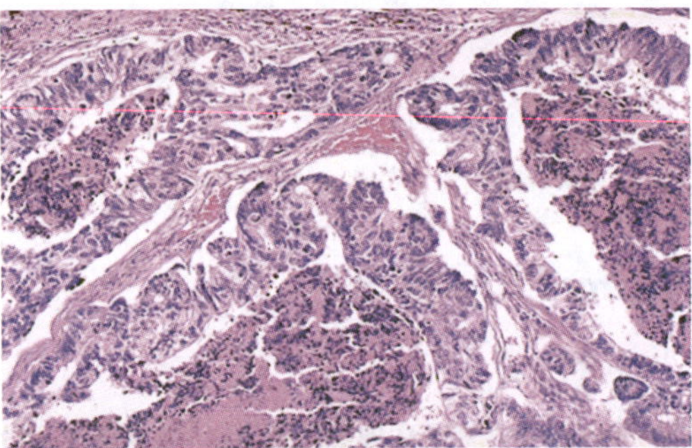

FIGURE 6.7 Microscopy of carcinoma colon

Carcinoma of the left side of colon (distal part) is usually annular, encircling lesions that produce "Napkin ring" constriction of the bowel. The margins of the napkin ring are classically heaped up, beaded and firm with ulcerated mid region. The lumen is markedly narrowed and the proximal bowel may be distended.

Microscopy: The microscopic picture of both right and left sided lesions is similar. It shows the classical picture of adenocarcinoma. It can be well differentiated with tall columnar tumor cells or poorly differentiated with anaplastic tumor cells. Mucin is produced in many tumors. Many other tumors may show a signet ring appearance (Fig. 6.7).

Spread: All colorectal carcinomas metastatize through the gut wall into the lymphatics and blood vessels. It can involve the regional lymph nodes, liver, lungs and bones.

CHAPTER 7

Liver, Gallbladder and Pancreas

LIVER

Normal Structure

Anatomy

The liver weighs around 1400 to 1600 g in males and 1200 to 1400 g in females. It has right and left lobes and is enclosed by a layer of connective tissue called *Glisson's capsule.* On its inferior surface are the gallbladder and extra-hepatic bile ducts. Liver has dual blood supply. The portal vein brings venous blood and the hepatic artery supplies arterial blood to the liver. The venous drainage from the liver is into the right and left hepatic veins, which drains into inferior vena cava (Fig. 7.1).

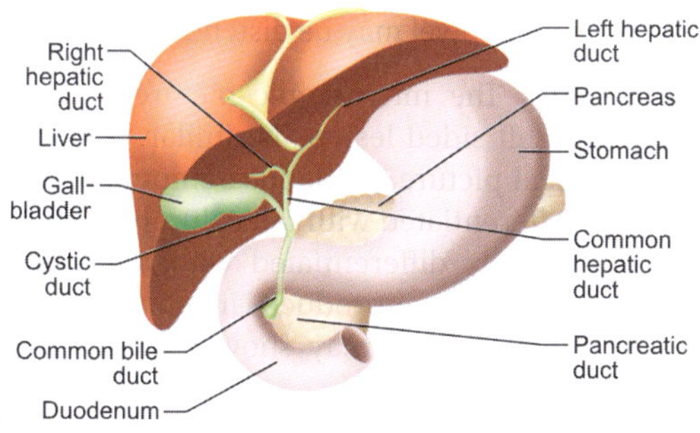

FIGURE 7.1 Diagrammatic representation of hepatobiliary system

Normal Histology

The hepatic parenchyma is made-up of hexagonal lobules each of which has a central tributary from the hepatic vein, commonly called central vein and at the periphery the portal triads consisting of bile duct, portal vein and hepatic artery. The blood filled sinusoids are seen between the cords of hepatocytes and are lined by discontinuous endothelial cells and Kupffer cells. The hepatocytes are polygonal cells with a round nucleus and a prominent nucleolus (Fig. 7.2).

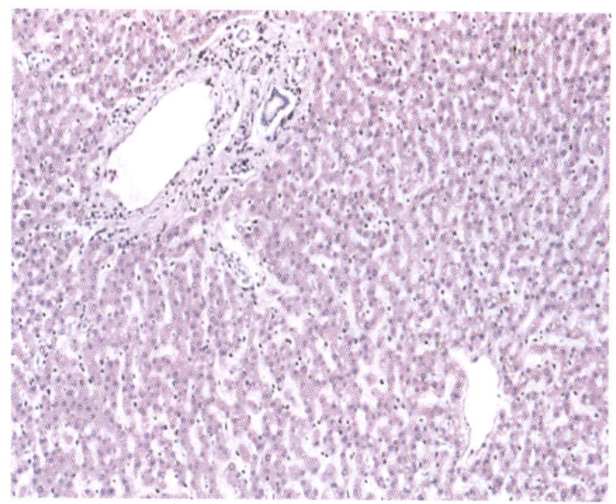

FIGURE 7.2 Histology of liver

GALLBLADDER

Normal Structure

Anatomy

The gallbladder is a pear shaped organ, 9 cm in length and has a volume of around 50 mL. It has fundus, body and neck. The neck tapers into cystic duct.

Normal Histology

The gallbladder lacks muscularis mucosae and submucosa. The wall of the gallbladder is composed of four layers. They are:

1. Mucosal layer which has a single layer of tall columnar epithelium.
2. Smooth muscle layer with inner longitudinal, middle oblique and outer circular muscle bundles.
3. Perimuscular layer, which is made of connective tissue with interspersed fat cells.
4. Serosal layer (Fig. 7.3).

PANCREAS

Normal Structure

Anatomy

The pancreas is an elongated structure about 15 cm in length. It is divided into head, body and tail.

Normal Histology

The exocrine pancreas constitutes 80 to 85 percent of the total gland while the remaining part is endocrine pancreas. The exocrine part is divided into lobules composed of numerous acini. These acini are lined by pyramid shaped columnar epithelial cells. These secretory epithelial cells have microvilli and their apical portion contain zymogen granules. The lobules are separated by thin fibrous septa which contain blood vessels, lymphatics, nerves and ducts (Fig. 7.4).

Jaundice

Jaundice or icterus is the yellowish discoloration of the skin or sclerae. It is due to increase in the serum bilirubin. The normal serum bilirubin concentration ranges from 0.2–0.8 mg/dL. Jaundice is clinically appreciable when the total serum bilirubin exceeds 2 mg/dL.

Jaundice is divided into:

- *Prehepatic or hemolytic jaundice*: Here *unconjugated* hyperbilirubinemia is seen. Jaundice is due to increased bilirubin caused by hemolysis.
- *Hepatic jaundice*: Here jaundice is due to increased bilirubin production, decreased hepatic uptake or decreased hepatic conjugation. Here again *unconjugated* hyperbilirubinemia is seen.

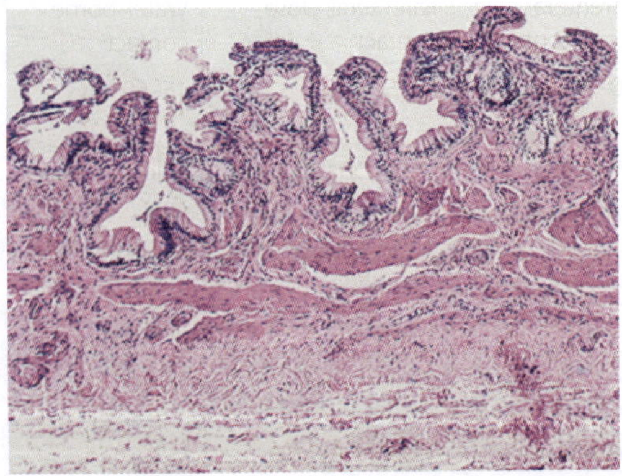

FIGURE 7.3 Histology of gallbladder

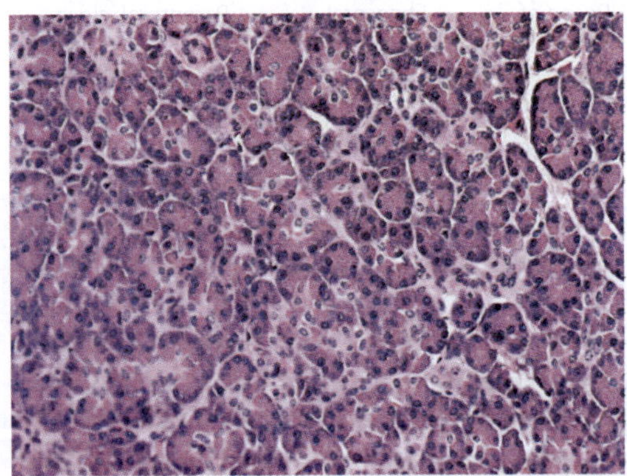

FIGURE 7.4 Histology of pancreas

- *Posthepatic or obstructive jaundice*: Here jaundice is due to intrahepatic or extrahepatic cholestasis or obstruction. This causes *conjugated* hyperbilirubinemia.

  Bilirubin pigment has high affinity for elastic tissue and hence is readily noticeable in tissues like sclera.

VIRAL HEPATITIS

Viral hepatitis is the infection of the liver caused by hepatotropic viruses, such as hepatitis A, B, C, D and E viruses. All these viruses are RNA viruses except hepatitis B virus which is a DNA virus (Table 7.1).

Hepatitis A Virus

Hepatitis A virus (HAV) is a small, 27 nm diameter icosahedral nonenveloped, single stranded RNA virus. The disease is associated with poor hygiene, over-crowding and poor sanitation. It is self-limiting. Chronic carriers have not been identified. IgM anti-HAV antibody appears in the serum at the onset of symptoms. IgG anti-HAV antibody is detected after IgM antibody and gives life-long immunity.

Hepatitis B Virus

Electron microscopic study reveals large 42 nm Dane particles representing the intact hepatitis B virus (HBV). Dane particle is spherical with a diameter of 42 nm, partially single stranded and partially double stranded. It has an outer envelope and an inner hexagonal core measuring 27 nm and containing double stranded DNA, which is associated with DNA polymerase. The surface envelope contains hepatitis B surface antigen (HBsAg) and the inner core has hepatitis core antigen (HBcAg) and another antigen called HBeAg (Fig. 7.5).

The disease spreads by transfusion of infected blood or blood products, needle pricks, accidental cuts or by sexual contact.

TABLE 7.1 Characteristics of hepatic viruses

Feature	*Hepatitis A virus (HAV)*	*Hepatitis B virus (HBV)*	*Hepatitis C virus (HCV)*	*Hepatitis D virus (HDV)*	*Hepatitis E virus (HEV)*
Type of virus	Single stranded RNA	Double stranded DNA	Single stranded RNA	Single stranded RNA (defective)	Single stranded RNA
Morphology	Icosahedral, nonenveloped	Double shelled, enveloped	Enveloped	Enveloped, defective replication	Icosahedral, nonenveloped
Route of transmission	Feco-oral	Parenteral, close contact and sexual	Parenteral, close contact	Parenteral, close contact	Water-borne contact
Incubation period	15–45 days	30–180 days	20–90 days	30–50 days	15–60 days
Severity	Mild	Occasionally severe	Moderate	Occasionally severe	Mild
Chronic hepatitis	None	Occasional (10%)	Common (80%)	5% for coinfection, 70% for super infection	None
Carrier state	None	<1%	<1%	1–10%	unknown
Hepatocellular carcinoma	No	+	+	±	None
Prognosis	Excellent	Worse with age	Moderate	Acute–good Chronic–bad	Good

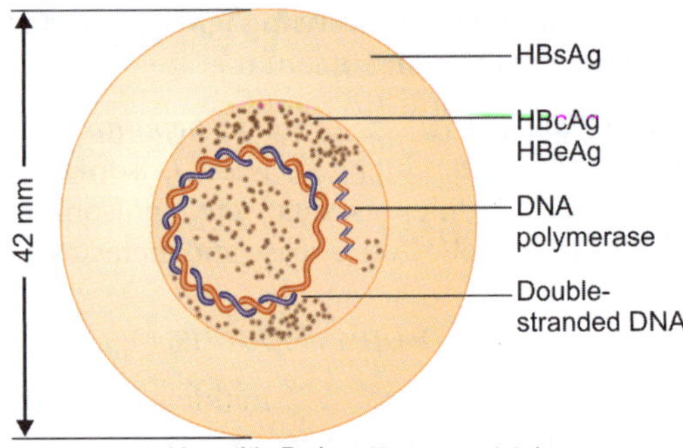

FIGURE 7.5 Diagrammatic representation of dane particle

Immunological Markers

- HBsAg appears early in the blood after about 6 weeks of infection and disappears by 3 to 6 months. Its presence even after 6 months implies a carrier state
- Anti-HBs antibody appears late, about 3 months after the onset
- HBeAg is present during an acute attack. Its persistence beyond 10 weeks implies chronic liver disease and carrier state
- Anti-HBe antibody appears after HBeAg disappears. Seroconversion from HBeAg to Anti-HBe during acute illness implies resolution of infection
- HBcAg cannot be detected in the blood
- Anti-HBc antibody can be detected in the serum during preicteric phase
- HBV-DNA detected by molecular methods is the sensitive index of hepatitis B infection.

Hepatitis D Virus

Hepatitis Delta virus is a small single stranded RNA particle with a diameter of 36 nm. It is highly infectious and can cause hepatitis in any HBsAg positive host. Hepatitis D develops when there is concomitant hepatitis B infection. When both infections occur simultaneously, it is called *co-infection*. When HDV infects a chronic HBsAg carrier, it is called *super infection*.

Hepatitis C Virus

Hepatitis C virus is a single stranded, enveloped RNA virus with 30 to 60 nm diameter. Hepatitis C infection is acquired by blood transfusions, blood products, hemodialysis, needle pricks and accidental cuts. HCV-RNA can be detected by PCR technique within a few days after exposure to HCV infection, much before the appearance of anti-HCV antibody and persists during the infection.

Hepatitis E Virus

Hepatitis E virus is a single stranded 32 to 34 nm, icosahedral nonenveloped virus. Hepatitis E is an enterically transmitted virus. The infection is acquired by contaminated water. HEV infection in pregnant woman show high mortality.

Clinicopathological Spectrum

- *Carrier state*
  - Asymptomatic healthy carrier—does not suffer from the disease.
  - Asymptomatic carrier with chronic disease.
- *Asymptomatic infection*—serum transaminases and antibodies are elevated.
- *Acute hepatitis*—it has four phases.
  - *Incubation period*—varies for different viruses
  - *Preicterus phase*—patient experiences fatigue, malaise, nausea, vomiting, anorexia, arthralgia, headache and low grade fever.
  - *Icteric phase (1-4 weeks)*—In this phase, clinical jaundice is seen along with constitutional symptoms, dark urine, clay stools, pruritus, loss of weight, abdominal discomfort and enlarged tender liver.
  - *Posticteric phase*—recovery is seen. Hepatitis B and C may show chronicity.
- *Chronic hepatitis*—fatigue, malaise, loss of appetite are seen. Some cases show enlarged tender liver and also mild splenomegaly. Some do not progress for several years

whereas others may show rapid evolution into cirrhosis.

- *Fulminant hepatitis*—most severe form with rapid progress to hepatocellular failure.

Pathology in Acute Hepatitis

Gross: Liver gets enlarged. It becomes soft and greenish.

Microscopy: Based on microscopy we can differentiate one viral infection from other. The virus invades the hepatocytes and causes their destruction. Many other morphological changes are associated with this.

- *Hepatocellular injury:* The injured hepatocytes show granules and vacuolization in their cytoplasm and appear swollen (*ballooning degeneration*). The necrotic cell remains as an acidophilic mass called *Councilman body or acidophil body*.
- *Inflammatory infiltrate:* Mononuclear cells infiltrate the portal tract and also can spread to hepatic lobules.
- *Kupfer cell hyperplasia:* Kupfer cells increase and phagocytose cellular debris, bile pigment and lipofuscin granules.
- *Bile stasis:* Intracytoplasmic bile pigment granules can be seen.
- *Regeneration:* Surviving hepatocytes undergo regeneration.

Some nonviral causes of acute hepatitis are: Drugs like acetaminophen, NSAID, isoniazid, halothane, antidepressants, etc. poisoning, hypoxia, alcoholic liver disease and metastasis.

Pathology in Chronic Hepatitis

- *Piecemeal necrosis:* It is nothing but periportal destruction of hepatocytes.
- *Portal tract lesions:* Inflammatory cells seen in the portal tract are lymphocytes, plasma cells and macrophages (triaditis).
- *Changes in the hepatocytes:* In hepatitis C infection moderate fatty change is seen. Hepatitis B infection causes ground-glass hepatocytes. More severe injury causes bridging necrosis (portal tract to portal tract, portal tract to central vein, and central vein to central vein).
- *Bridging fibrosis:* Initially, there is only periportal fibrosis, which later shows bridging between portal tract to portal tract and portal tract to central vein. In the end stage, there is total destruction of the lobular architecture. Nodules are formed and this is referred to as postnecrotic cirrhosis (Fig. 7.6).

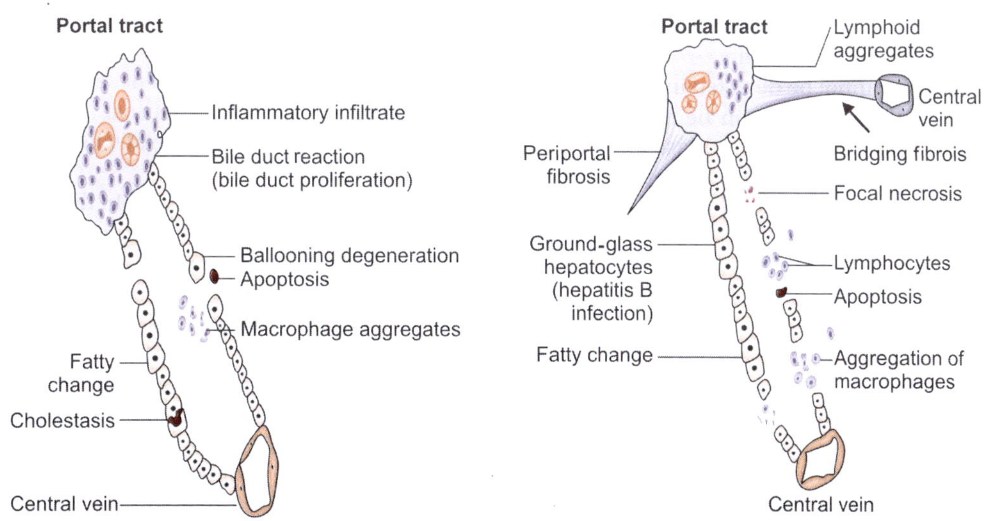

FIGURE 7.6 Diagrammatic representation of acute and chronic hepatitis

CIRRHOSIS OF LIVER

Cirrhosis is the irreversible end stage of chronic liver disease and is characterized by:

- Fibrosis—bridging septa in the form of delicate bands or broad scars.
- Nodules created by regeneration of hepatocytes encircled by fibrosis.
- Hepatic parenchymal architecture is disrupted.

Major causes of cirrhosis are:

- Alcoholic liver disease
- Viral hepatitis B, C and D
- Biliary diseases
- Primary hemochromatosis
- Wilson's disease
- α1- antitrypsin deficiency
- Cryptogenic cirrhosis
- Drugs
- Idiopathic.

Pathogenesis

Cirrhosis is initiated by hepatocellular necrosis. There occurs destruction of hepatocytes, which leads to collapse of normal lobular hepatic parenchyma followed by fibrosis around the necrotic liver cells and there is formation of regenerative nodules.

Pathology

Gross

The surface of the liver is studded with diffuse nodules, which vary little in size. Cirrhosis is divided into micronodular when the nodules are <3 mm in size and macronodular when they are >3 mm. It is sometimes of mixed type when nodules of both sizes are seen (Fig. 7.7).

Microscopy

- No lobular architecture is identified.
- Fibrous septa that divide the hepatic parenchyma extend from portal tract to central vein or portal tract to portal tract or both. As the scarring increases, the fibrous septa become thicker (Fig. 7.8).

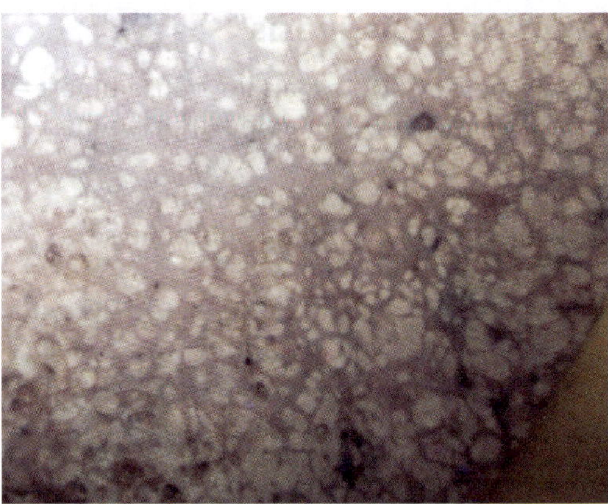

FIGURE 7.7 Gross photograph of cirrhosis liver

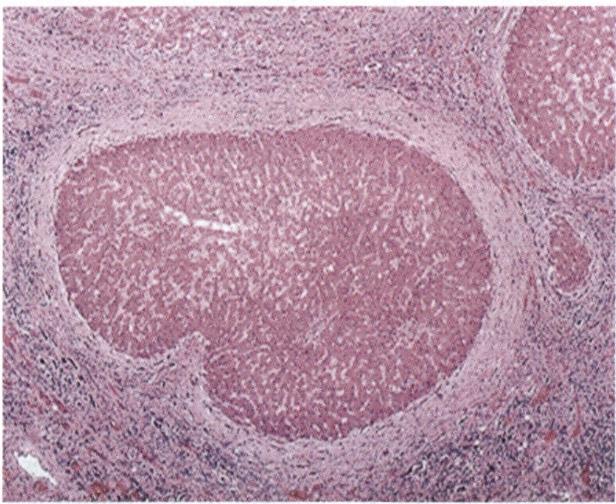

FIGURE 7.8 Microscopy of cirrhosis liver

Clinical Features

It may be asymptomatic for years. Finally cirrhosis presents with weight-loss, weakness, anorexia and osteoporosis. Once portal hypertension develops due to fibrosis of liver and impedance in blood supply, ascites, splenomegaly and portosystemic anastomoses develop. The causes of death in cirrhosis are hepatic failure, hepatocellular carcinoma and complications of portal hypertension.

Laboratory Diagnosis

- Elevated SGOT (aspartate transaminase—AST) and SGPT (alanine transaminase—ALT)
- Elevated γ glutamyl transpeptidase
- Elevated serum alkaline phosphatase
- Hyperbilirubinemia
- Hypoproteinemia with reversal of A:G ratio
- Prolonged PT and APTT time
- Anemia.

LIVER ABSCESS

The abscesses of the liver are of most commonly bacterial origin (pyogenic). The amebic liver abscess and the abscess due to hydatid disease and actinomycosis are rare.

Pyogenic Liver Abscess

The most common organisms involved are *E. coli, Pseudomonas, Klebsiella, Enterobacter* and a number of anaerobic organisms.

Pathology

Gross

The abscess may be single or multiple. They may measure 1 cm or more in diameter. These abscesses are more common in the right lobe of the liver and generally have a thick fibrous capsule (Fig. 7.9).

Microscopy

It shows small neutrophilic abscesses and areas of necrosis.

Clinical Features

The patient presents with severe abdominal pain in the right upper quadrant with fever and jaundice.

Laboratory Diagnosis

Elevated serum alkaline phosphatase, hypoalbuminemia and increase in the leukocytes in the blood.

Amebic Liver Abscess

They are caused by the spread of the organism *Entamoeba histolytica* from the intestinal lesions to the liver. The trophozoites of these amebae invade the colonic mucosa to form flask shaped ulcers and enter portal venous system to come to liver.

Pathology

Gross

These abscesses are usually single and are located in the right lobe, posterosuperior portion. The size of the abscesses may vary. The center of the abscess show reddish brown, thick pus resembling *anchovy sauce.* The wall of the abscess consists of irregular necrotic liver tissue.

Microscopy

It shows necrosis of the hepatocytes, leukocytes, red blood cells and debris. Amebae may be found in the liver tissue at the margin of the abscess.

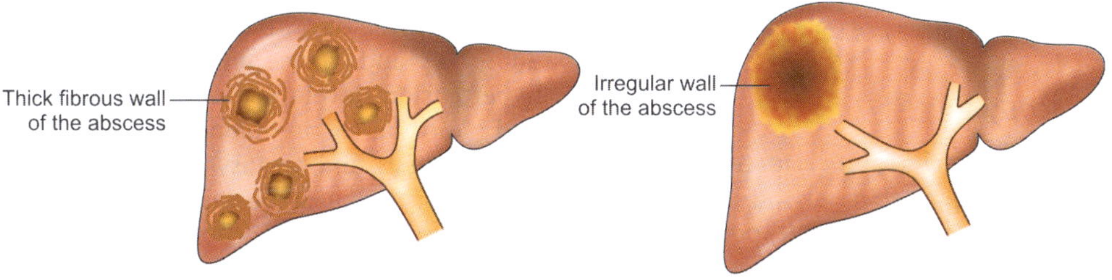

FIGURE 7.9 Diagrammatic representation of pyogenic abscess and amebic liver abscess

Clinical Features

The patient presents with pain and tenderness in the right-upper quadrant of the abdomen with intermittent low-grade fever. The patients may give history of amebic dysentery in the past.

Laboratory Diagnosis

Hemagglutination test is done. Cysts of *E. histolytica* are found in stools of some patients.

GALLBLADDER

Cholecystitis

Cholecystitis is the inflammation of the gallbladder. It is divided into acute and chronic.

Acute Cholecystitis

Based on the etiology it is classified into:

- Acute calculous cholecystitis (90%)—here inflammation occurs due to gallstone obstructing the neck of the gallbladder. Later secondary bacterial infection occurs. The organisms involved are *E. coli* and *Streptococcus faecalis*.
- Acute acalculous cholecystitis (10%)—here the inflammation occurs due to various causes like severe sepsis, dehydration, nonbiliary surgery, torsion of gallbladder and diabetes mellitus. Rare causes are cholera and salmonellosis.

Pathology

Gross

The gallbladder is distended and tense. The serosal surface is seen coated with fibrinous exudates with congestion and hemorrhage. The lumen when cut open may contain pus with bile. In calculous cholecystitis, a stone can be seen impacted in the neck or seen obstructing the cystic duct. When the lumen is filled with purulent exudates, it is called *empyema of the gallbladder*.

Microscopy

Neutrophilic exudates, congestion and edema are seen in the wall of the gallbladder.

Clinical Features

The patients present with severe pain in the upper abdomen, mild jaundice and fever. The gallbladder is tender.

Laboratory Diagnosis

Leukocytosis and neutrophilia is seen in the blood.

Chronic Cholecystitis

This is the most common type. It is almost always associated with cholelithiasis (gallstones). In some repeated attacks of acute cholecystitis leads to chronic cholecystitis.

Pathology

Gross

The gallbladder is contracted but may sometimes be normal or even enlarged. The wall of the gallbladder is thickened. The lumen may show multiple mixed stones.

Microscopy

Mucosa show congestion and thickening. Mucosa, sometimes, penetrate deep into the wall up to muscularis layer to form *Rokitansky-Aschoff sinuses*. Chronic inflammatory cells like lymphocytes, plasma cells and macrophages are present in the lamina propria and subserosal layer. Fibrosis is evident in subepithelial and subserosal layers.

Clinical Features

The patient is usually a fat, fertile, female of forty years with abdominal discomfort after a fatty meal. Dull ache in the right-upper quadrant of abdomen, nausea and flatulence are common.

Laboratory Diagnosis

Cholecystography is done to visualize the gallstones.

TUMORS OF LIVER

Hepatocellular Carcinoma

It is more common in men and at the age of around 50 years.

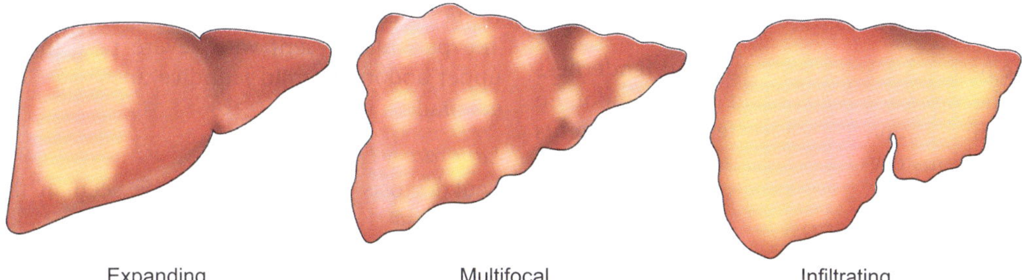

FIGURE 7.10 Diagrammatic representation of types of gross appearance in hepatocellular carcinoma

Etiology

- Hepatitis B and hepatitis C infection
- Cirrhosis
- Alcoholic liver disease
- Hemochromatosis
- Aflatoxin—produced by *Aspergillus flavus*.
- Metabolic liver disease
- Miscellaneous—schistosomiasis, tobacco smoking and α-antitrypsin deficiency.

Pathology

Gross

There are three patterns of growth:

1. *Expanding type*—usually seen as a single, yellow brown mass in the right lobe of the liver.
2. *Multifocal type*—multiple masses scattered throughout the liver.
3. *Infiltrating type*—diffuse infiltrating mass (Fig. 7.10).

Microscopy

Neoplastic hepatocytes are arranged in the trabecular, acinar and glandular, compact and patterns in a richly vascular stroma. Each neoplastic hepatocyte show vesicular nuclei with prominent nucleoli. The cytoplasm is granular and eosinophilic.

There is a variant of hepatocellular carcinoma called fibrolamellar carcinoma which is more common in young people of both sexes. It, usually, presents as a single mass and occurs in the absence of cirrhosis and has a better prognosis (Fig. 7.11).

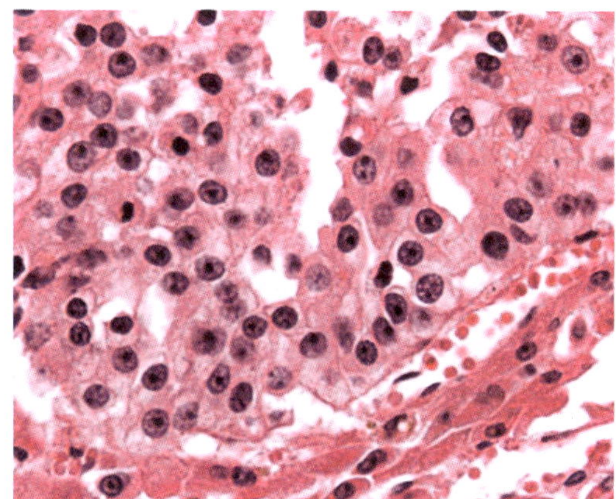

FIGURE 7.11 Microscopy of hepatocellular carcinoma

Clinical Features

The common features are enlarged tender liver, fever, fatigue, malaise and jaundice.

Laboratory Diagnosis

High levels of alpha feto protein (AFP) are seen in many patients.

Spread

The hepatocellular carcinoma (HCC) show both intrahepatic and extrahepatic spread. In intrahepatic spread, it causes multiple metastases in the liver. Extrahepatic spread occurs through blood to regional lymph nodes, lung, brain and bones.

TUMORS OF THE GALLBLADDER

Carcinoma Gallbladder

It is more common in women than men with a peak incidence in 7th decade. It is a slow growing tumor.

Etiology

Long-standing calculi, chemical carcinogens like nitrosamines, genetic causes and miscellaneous causes like previous biliary tract surgery and inflammatory bowel disease.

Pathology

The most common site is the fundus followed by neck of the gallbladder.

Gross

It is of two types:

1. Infiltrating type—irregular diffuse thickening of the gallbladder wall.
2. Fungating type—irregular, friable cauliflower like growth.

Microscopy

It is usually an adenocarcinoma (90%).

Clinical Features

Symptoms are seen very late in the disease. Symptomatic cases show pain, jaundice, weight-loss and anorexia.

Spread

It spreads to adjacent liver and through lympho-hematogenous route spreads to lung, peritoneum and gastrointestinal tract.

TUMORS OF THE EXOCRINE PANCREAS

Carcinoma Pancreas

It is common in males than females and the incidence increases after the age of 60 years.

Etiology

The etiological agents are smoking, diet with high caloric content, chemical carcinogens like nitrosamines, benzidine and beta naphthylamines, diabetes mellitus, chronic pancreatitis.

Pathology

Gross

The common locations are head, body and tail in the decreasing order of frequency. It presents as an irregular, grayish white mass with infiltrating margins.

Microscopy

Most arise from the ductal epithelium. It is most commonly an adenocarcinoma with variable differentiation. Other forms are adenoacanthoma and acinic cell carcinoma.

Clinical Features

It presents with obstructive jaundice causing dark urine, clay colored stools, pruritus. Other features are abdominal pain, weightloss, malaise, cachexia and migratory thrombophlebitis (Trousseau's syndrome).

CHAPTER 8

Kidney and Urinary Tract

KIDNEY

Anatomy

Kidney is a bean-shaped organ located in the retroperitoneum. It is surrounded by a thin fibrous capsule. On the medial aspect, at the midpoint, each kidney has a hilum, wherein the artery, vein, lymphatics and the ureter are located.

On cut section, kidney shows an outer cortex and inner medulla. The cortex is formed by the collecting tubules, ascending limbs and straight portions of the proximal convoluted tubules. The medulla is composed of several cone-shaped renal pyramids. The apex of each pyramid is called the *papilla* (Fig. 8.1).

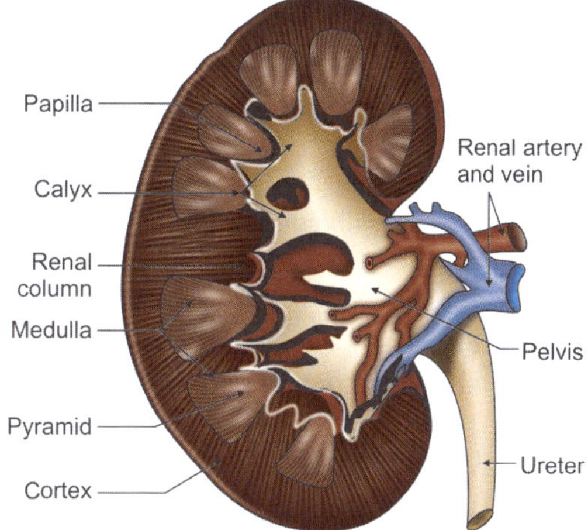

FIGURE 8.1 Diagrammatic representation of cut section of the kidney

Histology: Each renal parenchyma has approximately one million nephrons (Fig. 8.2).

Parts of each nephron:
- Glomerulus
- Proximal convoluted tubule
- Loop of Henle
- Distal convoluted tubule
- Collecting ducts.

PATHOLOGY (TABLE 8.1)

Acute Glomerulonephritis

Acute glomerulonephritis is a group of glomerular diseases, where in there is inflammation of the glomerulus, which give rise to characteristic clinical syndrome of nephritis. This nephritic syndrome presents with hematuria (blood in urine), RBC casts in urine, azotemia, oliguria (reduced urine output), mild proteinuria, edema and moderate hypertension.

ACUTE PROLIFERATIVE GLOMERULONEPHRITIS

This disease is characterized by diffuse proliferation of glomerular cells along with leukocytic infiltrate.

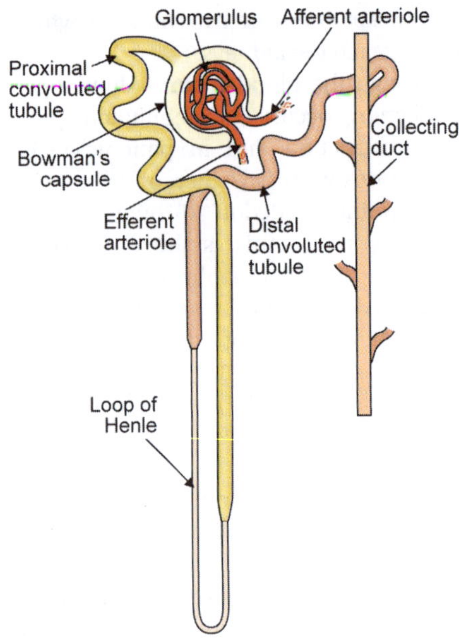

FIGURE 8.2 Diagrammatic representation of the parts of a nephron

Poststreptococcal Glomerulonephritis

This type of glomerular disease usually follows one to four weeks after a streptococcal infection of the throat or skin. It is seen commonly in children aged between 6 and 10 years of age.

Etiopathogenesis

Poststreptococcal glomerular disease is an immunologically mediated disease. The antibodies formed against *Streptococcus* will form immune complexes with glomerular antigens and gets deposited in the glomerular basement membrane.

Morphology

The typical microscopic picture in this disease is enlarged, hypercellular glomeruli. The hypercellularity is due to infiltration by

TABLE 8.1 Different types of glomerulonephritis

Disease	*Clinical presentation*	*Microscopy*
Acute poststreptococcal glomerulonephritis	Acute nephritis	Hypercellular glomeruli; leukocytic infiltration
Goodpasture syndrome	Rapidly progressive glomerulonephritis	Hypercellular glomeruli; crescents
Idiopathic RPGN	Rapidly progressive glomerulonephritis	Cellular proliferation; focal necrosis; crescents
Membranous glomerulopathy	Nephrotic syndrome	Diffuse capillary wall thickening
Minimal change disease	Nephrotic syndrome	Normal light microscopy; loss of processes seen on electron microscopy
Focal segmental glomerulosclerosis	Nephrotic syndrome	Focal and segmental sclerosis; hyalinosis
Membranoproliferative glomerulonephritis	Nephrotic syndrome Hematuria Chronic renal failure	Mesangial proliferation; basement membrane thickening; splitting
IgA Nephropathy	Recurrent hematuria, proteinuria	Focal proliferative glomerulonephritis; mesangial widening
Chronic glomerulonephritis	Chronic renal failure	Hyalinized glomeruli

RPGN-Rapidly progressive glomerulonephritis; Nephrotic syndrome—It is a symptom complex with heavy proteinuria, albuminemia, generalized edema and lipidemia

leukocytes (neutrophils, monocytes), and proliferation of endothelial and mesangial cells. There may be interstitial edema and tubules often contain RBC casts (Fig. 8.3).

Clinical Features

In a typical case, the patient is usually a young child abruptly developing malaise, fever, nausea, oliguria and hematuria (cola-colored urine) one week after recovery from sore throat. The patient will have mild to moderate hypertension with mild proteinuria. Laboratory investigations will show increased anti-streptolysin O (ASLO) titers and cryoglobulin in the serum. Also there will be a reduction in serum C 3 component in the serum.

PYELONEPHRITIS

Pyelonephritis is a renal disease affecting the tubules, interstitium and renal pelvis.

It occurs in two forms:
1. Acute pyelonephritis
2. Chronic pyelonephritis.

Etiopathogenesis

The most important causative factors in pyelonephritis are gram negative bacilli such as *Escherichia coli, Proteus, Klebsiella* and *Enterobacter*. There are two routes by which the bacteria reach the kidneys:

1. Through the bloodstream—Hematogenous infection occurs in debilitated patients, in obstruction and in patients receiving immunosuppressive therapy.
2. Ascending infection through the lower urinary tract—This is the most common cause of pyelonephritis. The factors responsible for the causation are:
   - Colonization of distal urethra and introitus (in females) by coliform bacteria
   - Organisms gain entry into the urethra during catheterization or other instrumentation
   - The organisms multiply in the bladder either due to bladder dysfunction or increased residual urine volume.
   - Vesicoureteral reflux due to incompetent vesicoureteral valve, which allows the bacteria to ascend up to the kidney.
   - Intrarenal reflux allows for the establishment of infection throughout the renal parenchyma.

In the absence of vesicoureteral reflux, the infection remains localized to the urinary bladder causing cystitis, which is described in detail later.

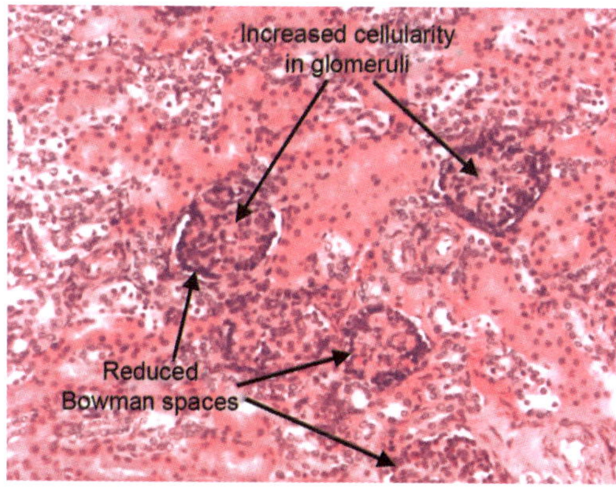

FIGURE 8.3 Microscopic picture of acute poststreptococcal glomerulonephritis

Acute Pyelonephritis

Acute pyelonephritis is an acute suppurative inflammation of the kidney caused by bacterial infection. It can be hematogenous or due to ascending infection in presence of vesicoureteral reflux.

Morphology

Microscopically, three important features are seen:
1. Patchy interstitial suppurative inflammation
2. Neutrophilic aggregates, within the tubules
3. Tubular necrosis.

Complications of acute pyelonephritis:
- Papillary necrosis
- Pyonephrosis
- Perinephric abscess.

Clinical Features

Acute pyelonephritis is associated with one of the following predisposing conditions:

- Urinary tract obstruction
- Instrumentation
- Pregnancy
- Diabetes mellitus
- Immunosuppression and immuno-deficiency.

Clinically, it presents with a sudden onset of pain in the costovertebral region accompanied by high degree of fever and chills. There is dysuria, increased frequency and urgency of micturition. Urine analysis reveals leukocytes and pus casts. The diagnosis of causative bacteria is done by urine culture sensitivity.

Treatment with antibiotics and with plenty of fluids is curative.

Chronic Pyelonephritis

Chronic pyelonephritis is a chronic interstitial renal disease in which chronic tubulointerstitial inflammation and renal scarring are associated with pathologic involvement of calyces and pelvis.

Types of Chronic Pyelonephritis

- Chronic reflux associated.
- Chronic obstructive pyelonephritis.

Morphology

Gross

The characteristic appearance of chronic pyelonephritis is irregular scarring of the kidney. If the involvement is bilateral, then it is asymmetrical. The hallmark of chronic pyelonephritis is coarse, discrete cortico-medullary scar overlying a dilated, blunted or a deformed calyx (Fig. 8.4).

Microscopy

The involvement is mainly seen in the tubules and the interstitium. Tubules can be dilated and are filled with eosinophilic colloid casts called thyroidization of tubules. Chronic interstitial infiltrate consisting of lymphocytes and plasma cells is seen. Glomeruli may be normal or may show periglomerular fibrosis. Fibrosis around the calyces is seen (Fig. 8.5).

Clinical Features

Chronic pyelonephritis is insidious in onset, presenting with clinical features of back pain, pyuria and fever.

If not treated, it can progress on to focal segmental glomerulosclerosis and chronic renal failure.

RENAL CALCULI/UROLITHIASIS (STONES)

Renal stone is a frequent cause of pain in the loin. Calculi can arise at any level in the urinary tract, frequently causing clinical symptoms such as pain (renal colic). They also predispose to renal infection.

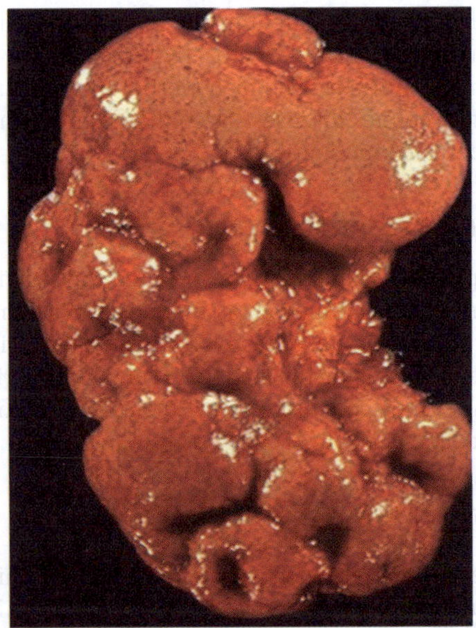

FIGURE 8.4 Gross picture of chronic pyelonephritis

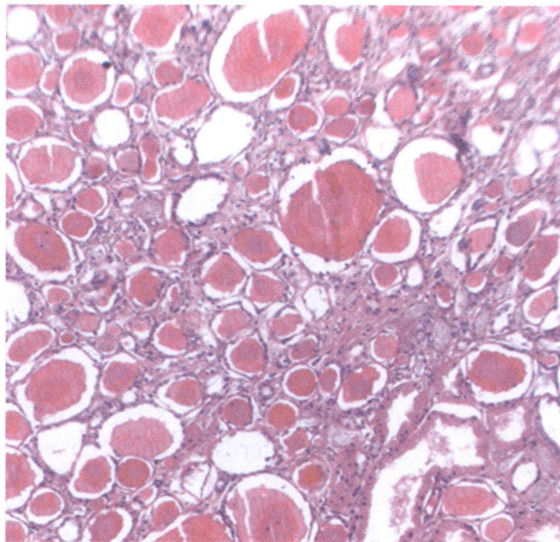

FIGURE 8.5 Microscopic picture of chronic pyelonephritis (note the thyroidization of tubules)

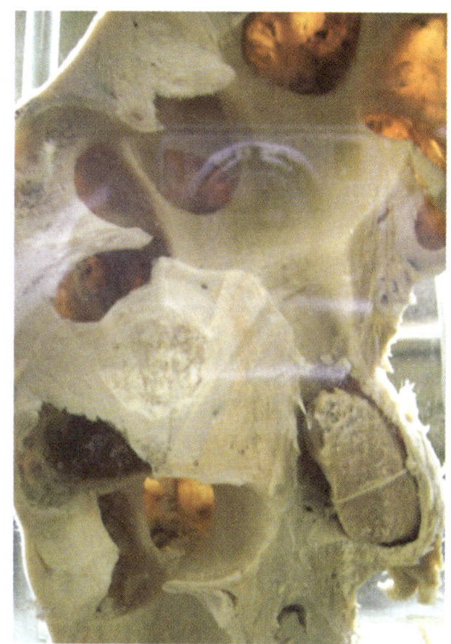

FIGURE 8.6 Gross picture of renal calculi

Types of Renal Calculi

Calcium Oxalate Stones

Seventy percent of renal stones are calcium containing, composed of calcium oxalate with or without calcium phosphate. They are usually associated with hypercalcemia or hypercalciuria caused by hyperparathyroidism, diffuse bone disease, sarcoidosis and other hypercalcemic states.

Triple Phosphate Stones

Triple phosphate stones also called the struvite stones, are composed of magnesium ammonium phosphate. These are associated with infection causing the stag horn calculi due to its shape. They constitute 15 to 20 percent of renal calculi.

Uric Acid Stones

These stones are seen in patients with uricemia, gout and rapid turnover state like leukemia. They constitute five to ten percent of renal stones.

Cystine Stones

Cystine stones seen in one to two percent of cases due to genetic deficiency in the absorption of cystine leading to cystinuria.

Increased concentrations of stone constituents, changes in urinary pH, decreased urine volume and bacteria play a role in the formation of stones (Fig. 8.6).

RENAL CELL CARCINOMA

Renal cell carcinoma constitutes about 85 percent of renal cancers in adults. It is usually seen in the old age between 60 and 70 years of age with a male preponderance. Risk factors include cigarette smoking, obesity, hypertension, unopposed estrogen therapy, exposure to petroleum products, heavy metals and asbestos. Most renal cell cancers are sporadic, but four percent are familial.

Morphology

Renal cell carcinoma usually arises from one of the poles, commonly the upper-pole of the kidney (Fig. 8.7).

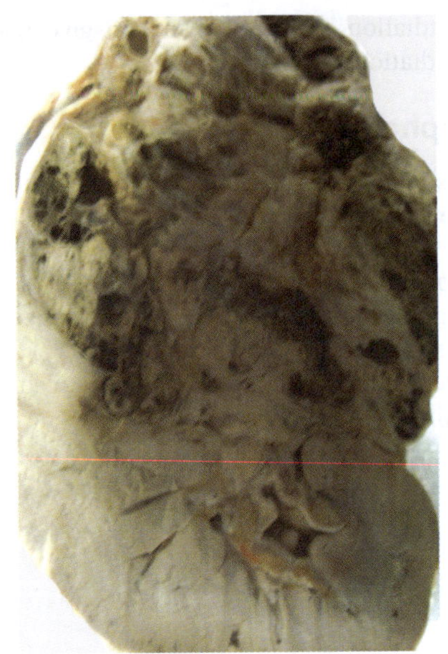

FIGURE 8.7 Gross picture of renal carcinoma

Types of Renal Cell Carcinoma

The classification is based on microscopy, cytogenetics and genetics.

Clear Cell Carcinoma

This is the most common type, accounting for 70 to 80 percent of primary renal cancers. Grossly, it is usually unilateral with spherical mass of varying size composed of bright yellow gray white tissue that distorts the renal outline. Areas of necrosis and hemorrhage are seen. Microscopically, the tumor cells grow in solid trabecular or tubular pattern. Individual tumor cells are round to polygonal with abundant clear to granular cytoplasm and atypical nucleus (Fig. 8.8).

Papillary Carcinoma

Accounts for 10 to 15 percent of renal cell cancers. Grossly, it can be multifocal and bilateral. They are typically hemorrhagic and cystic. It has a tendency to invade the renal vein and grow as solid column of cells within the vessel. Microscopically, it is composed of cuboidal or low columnar cells arranged in the form of papillae. Psammoma bodies may be present.

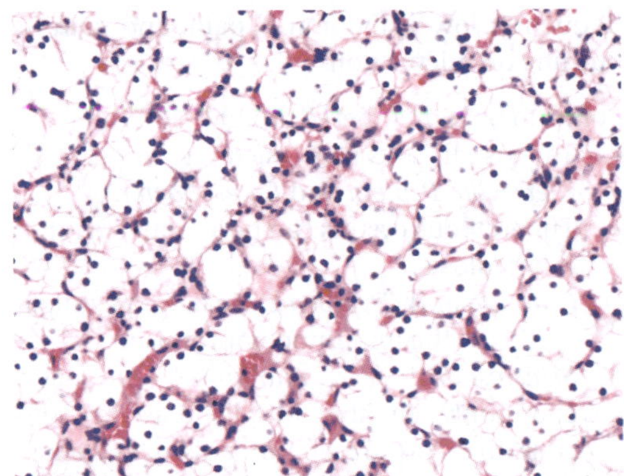

FIGURE 8.8 Microscopy of clear cell renal carcinoma

Chromophobe Renal Carcinoma

It constitutes five percent of renal cancers. Microscopically, it is made up of pale eosinophilic cells with a perinuclear halo arranged in solid sheets.

Clinical Features

The three diagnostic symptoms of renal cell cancer are costovertebral pain, palpable mass and hematuria. It is also associated with fever, malaise, weakness and weight loss. Most of the times, it will have metastasized widely at the time of diagnosis.

Prognosis

The average five year survival is 45 to 70 percent in absence of metastasis. With renal vein invasion, it is reduced to 10 to 20 percent. Nephrectomy is the treatment of choice.

CYSTITIS

Cystitis is the inflammation of the urinary bladder. The symptoms include urinary

frequency, lower abdominal pain, and pain or burning on micturition.

Points to be remembered about cystitis are:

- The usual causative bacteria are *E. coli, Klebsiella, Proteus* and *Enterobacter*.
- Tuberculous cystitis can be a sequel to renal tuberculosis.
- *Candida* and *Cryptococcus* can cause fungal cystitis in the immunocompromised.
- *Schistosoma haematobium* is seen commonly in the Middle East as the causative protozoan organism. Chemotherapeutic agents, such as cyclophosphamide and busulfan can produce hemorrhagic cystitis.
- Radiation of the bladder can give rise to radiation cystitis.

Morphology

Grossly, there is hyperemia of the mucosa, sometimes associated with exudate. When there is hemorrhage in the exudate, it is called hemorrhagic cystitis.

The accumulation of large amounts of pus results in suppurative cystitis.

Persistence of the infection leads to chronic cystitis.

CHAPTER 9

Male Genital System and Prostate

TESTIS: NORMAL STRUCTURE (FIG. 9.1)

Scrotal sac contains testicle and epididymis along with lower-end of spermatic cord and tunica vaginalis. The testis is composed of seminiferous tubules. Histologically these tubules contain many layers of cells. The cells are of two types:

1. Spermatogonia or germ cells—produce spermatocytes, spermatids and mature spermatozoa.
2. Sertoli cells—supportive cells to germ cells and they produce estrogen and androgen.

The stroma between these seminiferous tubules contains interstitial cells of Leydig. These Leydig cells have abundant cytoplasm and contain lipid and Reinke's crystals (Fig. 9.2).

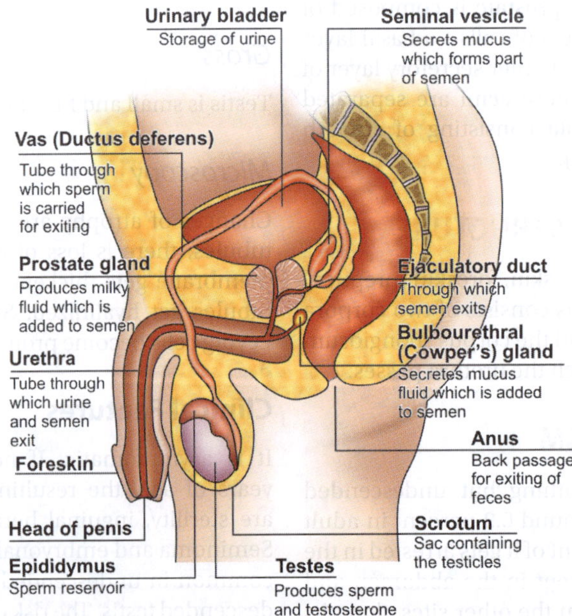

FIGURE 9.1: Diagrammatic representation of anatomy of male genital tract

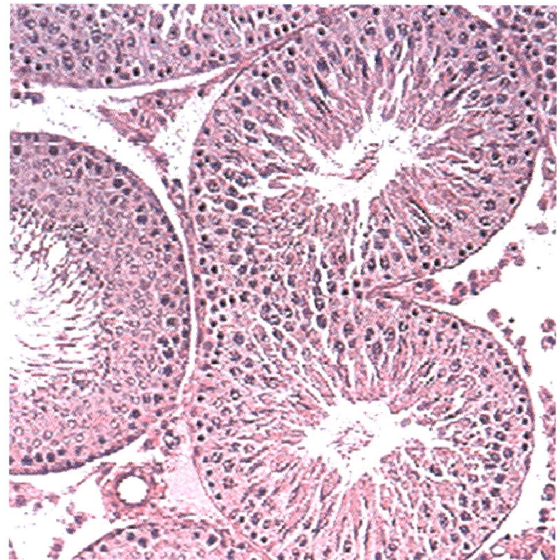

FIGURE 9.2: Histology of testis

PROSTATE: NORMAL STRUCTURE

The prostate gland in a normal adult weighs around 20 g. It has three lobes. They are two lateral lobes and a small median lobe.

Histologically, the prostate is composed of acini lined by two layers of cells—a basal layer of cuboidal cells and an inner secretory layer of tall columnar cells. These acini are separated by fibromuscular septa consisting of smooth muscle fibers (Fig. 9.3).

PENIS: NORMAL STRUCTURE

The penis is covered by skin, foreskin (prepuce) and mucosa. The penis consists of two corpora cavernosa, dorsally and the corpus spongiosum ventrally through which the urethra passes.

CRYPTORCHIDISM

Cryptorchidism is nothing but undescended testis. Incidence is around 0.2 percent in adult males. About 70 percent of it gets arrested in the inguinal ring, 25 percent in the abdomen and remaining 5 percent in the other sites along its descent from abdomen to scrotal sac.

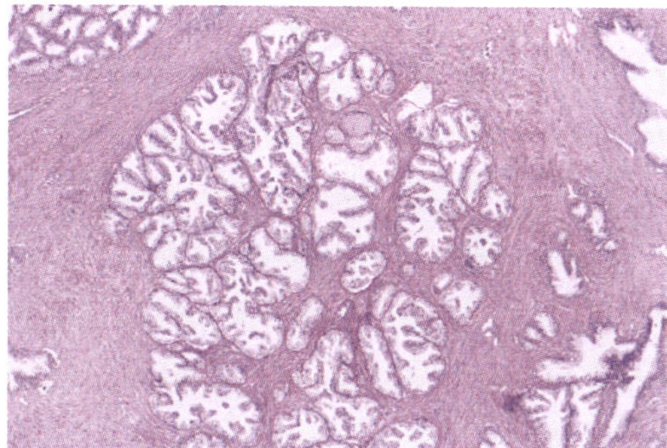

FIGURE 9.3: Histology of prostate

Etiology

In many of the cases, etiology is not known. Some known causes are short spermatic cord, narrow inguinal canal, maldevelopment of scrotum, trisomy 13 and deficient androgenic secretions.

Pathology

It is most commonly unilateral. In only 25 percent of the cases, it is bilateral.

Gross

Testis is small and fibrotic.

Microscopy

Changes of atrophy are seen. In seminiferous tubules, there is loss of germ cells, basement membrane gets thickened. In later stages, the tubules get hyalinized. Stroma increases and Leydig cells become prominent.

Clinical Features

It is asymptomatic. If not corrected by two years of age, the resulting adverse outcomes are sterility, inguinal hernia and malignancy. Seminoma and embryonal carcinoma are more common in undescended testis than normally descended testis. The risk of malignancy is more in the intra-abdominal location.

TESTICULAR ATROPHY

It is a regressive change that affects the testis and the causes are:

- Atherosclerotic narrowing of the blood vessels in old age
- Cryptorchidism
- End stage of orchitis
- Klinefelter syndrome
- Hypopituitarism
- Irradiation
- Female sex hormones given for a prolonged period in the treatment of carcinoma prostate
- Malnutrition and cachexia.

Morphology

Gross

The testis is small in size, firm and fibrotic.

Microscopy

Arrest in the development of germ cells with hyalinization of the tubules and thickening of the basement membrane. There is increase in the interstitial stroma with prominent Leydig cells (Fig. 9.4).

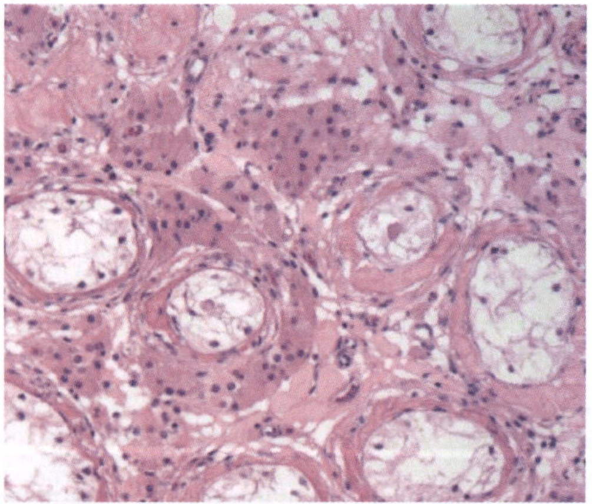

FIGURE 9.4: Microscopy of testicular atrophy

Clinical Features

When the condition is bilateral it causes sterility.

TESTICULAR TUMORS

They are divided into two main categories.

1. Germ cell tumors—derived from germ cells.
2. Nongerminal tumors—derived from stroma and sex cord.

Pathological classification of these tumors:

Germ Cell Tumors

- Seminoma
- Spermatocytic seminoma
- Embryonal carcinoma
- Yolk sac tumor (endodermal sinus)
- Choriocarcinoma
- Teratoma.

Sex Cord: Stromal Tumors

- Leydig cell tumor
- Sertoli cell tumor.

Seminoma

Seminomas are the most common germ cell tumor. It is more common in the thirties.

Morphology

Gross

Bulky masses with a homogeneous, gray white, lobulated cut surface usually devoid of hemorrhage or necrosis.

Microscopy

Sheets of uniform cells in lobules divided by delicate septa. The septa are usually infiltrated with lymphocytes. The seminoma cell is round, large and has a distinct cell membrane. Cytoplasm is clear with a central nucleus and one or more prominent nucleoli (Fig. 9.5).

The tumor cells stain positively for placental alkaline phosphatase.

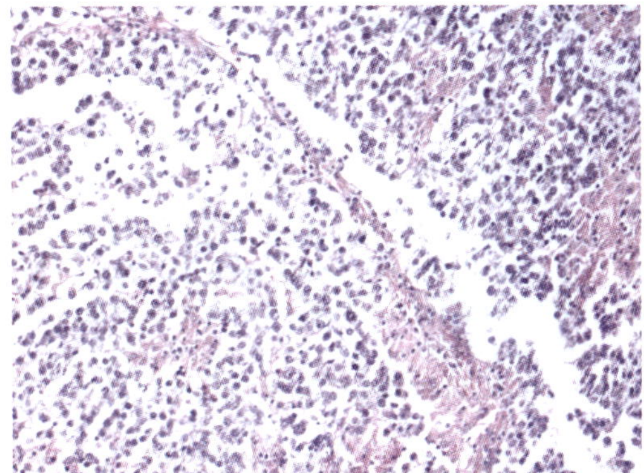

FIGURE 9.5: Microscopy of seminoma

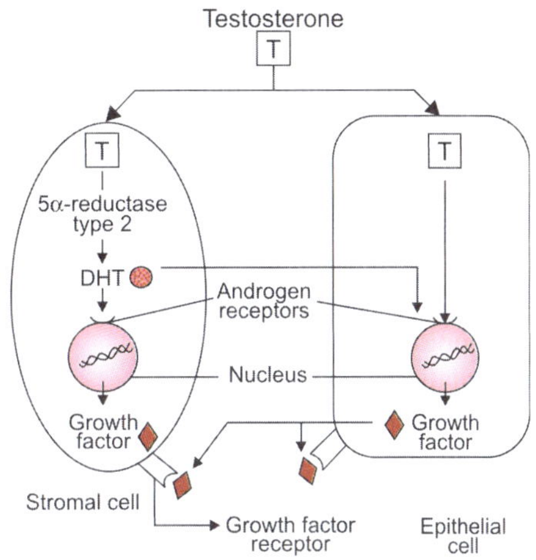

FIGURE 9.6: Diagrammatic representation of pathogenesis of prostatic hyperplasia

Clinical Features

Painless enlargement of the testis is seen in germ cell neoplasms. Any testicular mass should be considered neoplastic unless proved otherwise.

Spread

Lymphatic spread is common. It spreads to para-aortic lymph nodes, retroperitoneal, mediastinal and supraclavicular nodes.

Hematogenous spread occurs to lung, liver, brain and bones.

PROSTATE

Nodular Hyperplasia or Benign Prostatic Hyperplasia

It is very common in men after the age of 50 years. But symptoms are seen only in 5 to 10 percent of the cases. Benign prostatic hyperplasia (BPH) is characterized by hyperplasia of the stroma and the epithelial cells producing discrete nodules in the periurethral region of the prostate.

Etiopathogenesis

Prostatic enlargement is due to the action of androgens. Dihydrotestosterone (DHT) is a metabolite of testosterone and is the mediator of prostatic growth. It is synthesized in the prostate in the stromal cell by the action of the enzyme 5 α-reductase, type 2. This enzyme is principally located in the stromal cell. DHT once produced binds to nuclear androgen receptors of the stromal cell (autocrine type) and also of the epithelial cell (paracrine type), signals the transcription of growth factors that are mitogenic to epithelial and stromal cells.

Estrogen also play a role by making the cells more susceptible to the action of DHT (Fig. 9.6).

Morphology

Gross

Prostate is enlarged and the periurethral part (transition zone) is more commonly involved. It becomes nodular, smooth and firm. It weighs around 60 to 100 g (2–4 times its normal weight).

If it is predominantly an epithelial nodule, it is yellow, soft and milky fluid exudes from it. If it is mainly a fibromuscular (stromal) nodule, it is firm, homogeneous and does not exude any milky fluid. These enlargements compress the urethra into slit-like orifice.

Microscopy

Nodularity is a prominent feature. Glandular proliferation is seen in the form of small-large

to cystically dilated glands, lined by two layers, an inner columnar and an outer cuboidal or flattened layer. There might be intra-acinar papillary infoldings with delicate fibrovascular cores.

Stromal hyperplasia appears as spindle cells in aggregates. Other findings seen may be lymphocytic aggregates, areas of infarction and squamous metaplasia (Fig. 9.7).

Clinical Features

Symptoms are usually due to urethral obstruction and retention of urine in the bladder leading to hypertrophy of the bladder and cystitis. Patients present with frequency, nocturia, difficulty in urination, overflow dribbling and dysuria. In some cases, there is acute retention of urine requiring catheterization.

CARCINOMA PROSTATE

It is seen in men above 50 years.

Etiology

It is not quite clear. However, the role of androgens is supported by the fact that the orchiectomy causes arrest of metastatic prostatic carcinoma. There are some racial and geographic differences. Familial clustering and the carcinoma in first degree relatives suggest the possibility of genetic basis.

Pathology

Gross

In 95% of the cases the tumor is located in the peripheral zone. The prostate is firm and fibrous. It is enlarged, normal or smaller than normal.

Microscopy

The histological types are adenocarcinoma, transitional cell carcinoma, squamous cell carcinoma and undifferentiated carcinoma. But the most common type is adenocarcinoma and its characteristics are back-to-back arrangement of glands, loss of intra-acinar papillary convolutions and very little stroma. The glands are lined by a single layer of cells (cuboidal or low columnar). These tumor cells show varying degree of anaplasia. Invasion of intra-prostatic perineural spaces is common (Fig. 9.8).

Gleason's microscopic grading system is used to grade the prostatic cancers.

Clinical Features

In the initial stages, it is usually silent as it affects the peripheral part of the prostate and do not compress the urethra. By the time the symptoms appear, it is usually palpable on rectal examination. In symptomatic cases, the clinical features are urinary obstruction

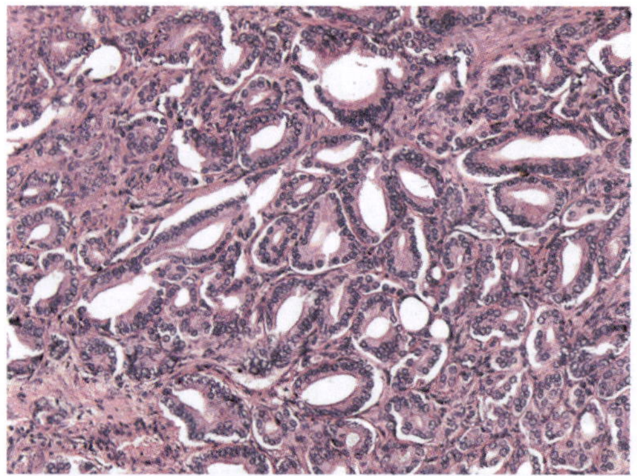

FIGURE 9.7: Microscopy of prostatic hyperplasia

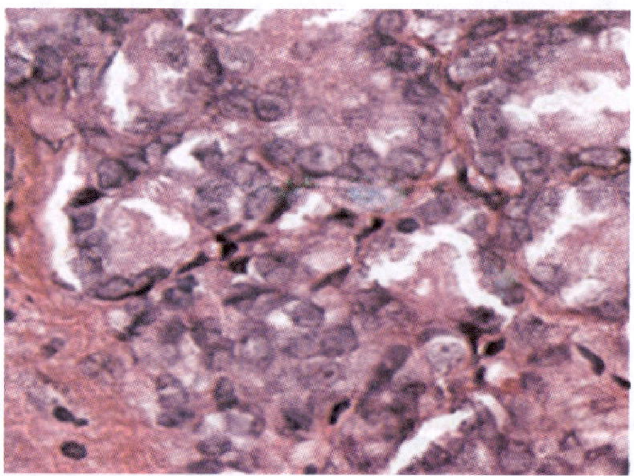

FIGURE 9.8: Microscopy of prostatic carcinoma

with dysuria, frequency, urinary retention and hematuria. In cases with skeletal metastasis, the patient complains of back pain.

Prostate specific antigen (PSA) is a protease enzyme secreted from prostatic cells and is detected by immunohistochemical method in the malignant prostatic epithelium as well as in the serum. In prostatic cancer, PSA increases considerably.

PSA assay is useful in deciding whether the metastasis originated from the prostate or not.

Prostatic acid phosphatase (PAP) is another enzyme secreted by prostatic epithelium. The serum level of this also increases in prostatic carcinoma which has metastasized.

Treatment of prostatic cancer is by surgery, radiotherapy and hormonal therapy.

CARCINOMA PENIS

Carcinoma of the penis is quite rare in Jews and Muslims, who have a ritual of circumcision. Circumcision gives protection against penile cancer due to prevention of accumulation of carcinogenic smegma. It is common between 45 and 65 years of age.

Pathology

Gross

The tumor is seen on frenum, prepuce, glans and coronal sulcus in the decreasing frequency. It is cauliflower-like, papillary, flat or ulcerating growth.

Microscopy

It is squamous cell carcinoma which is well differentiated to moderately differentiated.

Spread

It spreads to regional lymph nodes through lymphatics.

CHAPTER 10

Female Genital System and Breast

ANATOMY

The female reproductive system consists of vulva, vagina, uterus, fallopian tubes and ovaries. The primary function of this system is reproduction. Fertilization of ovum occurs in the fallopian tube. Implantation of the fertilized ovum occurs in the uterus (Fig. 10.1).

FIBROID/LEIOMYOMA

Fibroid is the commonly used term for benign tumor of the myometrium called leiomyoma.

Morphology

Gross

Leiomyomas are sharply circumscribed, discrete, round, firm, gray-white tumors with a whorled appearance on cut section (Fig. 10.2).

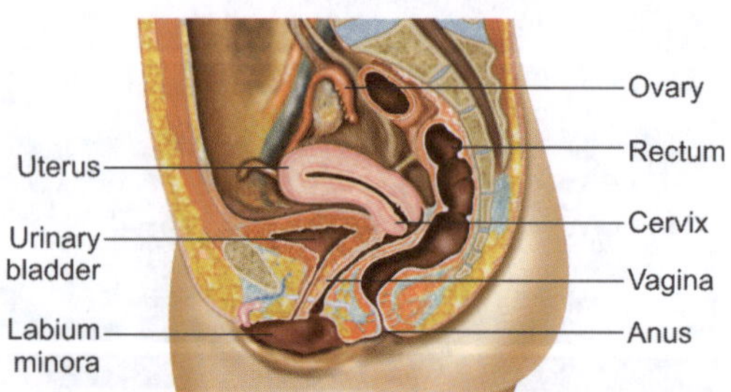

FIGURE 10.1 Anatomy of female genital tract

Leiomyomas are classified into various types based on the location:

a. *Submucosal*: Leiomyomas occurring just beneath the endometrium.
b. *Intramural*: Leiomyomas occurring within the myometrium.
c. *Subserosal*: Leiomyomas arising beneath the serosa.

Microscopy

On histologic examination, leiomyoma is composed of whorled bundles of smooth muscle cells. Usually individual muscle cells are uniform in size and shape and have the

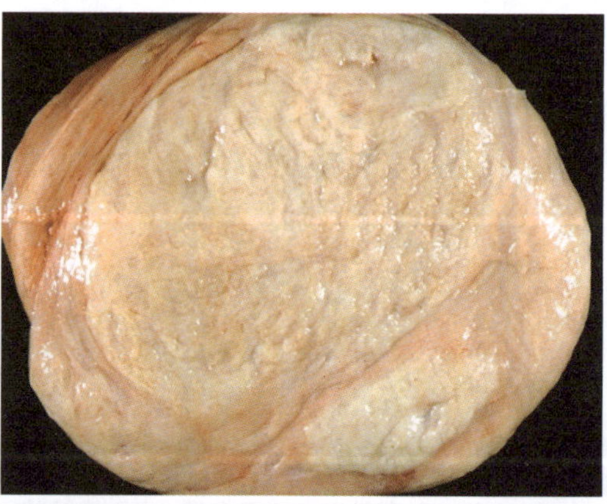

FIGURE 10.2 Gross appearance of leiomyoma

characteristic oval nucleus and long slender cytoplasmic processes. Mitotic figures are rare (Fig. 10.3).

Clinical Features

Some leiomyomas are asymptomatic while, others can cause a variety of symptoms like abnormal uterine bleeding, pain abdomen and impaired fertility. A submucosal leiomyoma can cause recurrent abortion or fetal malformation. Malignant transformation in a leiomyoma is extremely rare.

CARCINOMA OF THE ENDOMETRIUM

Endometrial carcinoma is the most common invasive cancer of the female genital tract.

Incidence

The peak incidence of endometrial carcinoma is in the 55–65 years of age. Higher frequency is seen with obesity, diabetes, hypertension and infertility.

Etiology and Pathogenesis

The endometrial carcinoma occurs in a background of estrogen stimulation and endometrial hyperplasia.

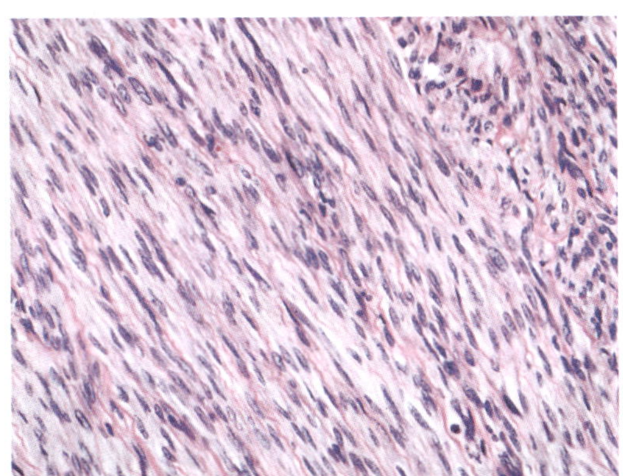

FIGURE 10.3 Microscopic picture of leiomyoma

Morphology

Gross

Grossly, it presents as either a localized polypoidal tumor or as a diffuse tumor involving the entire endometrial surface (Fig. 10.4).

Microscopy

On histologic examination, most endometrial carcinomas are adenocarcinomas characterized by well-defined gland formation. It can be divided into well differentiated, moderately differentiated and poorly differentiated (Fig. 10.5).

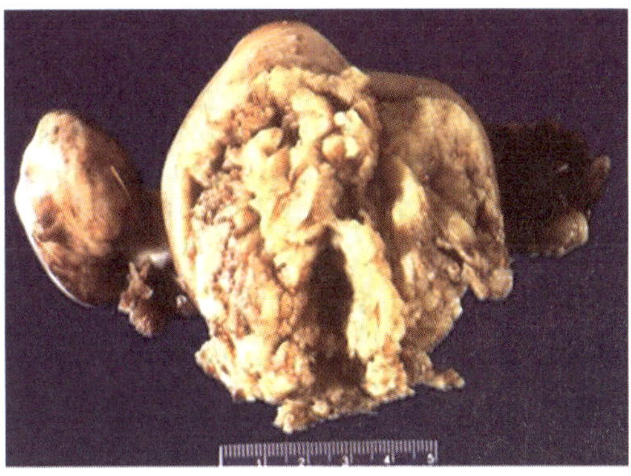

FIGURE 10.4 Gross picture of endometrial carcinoma

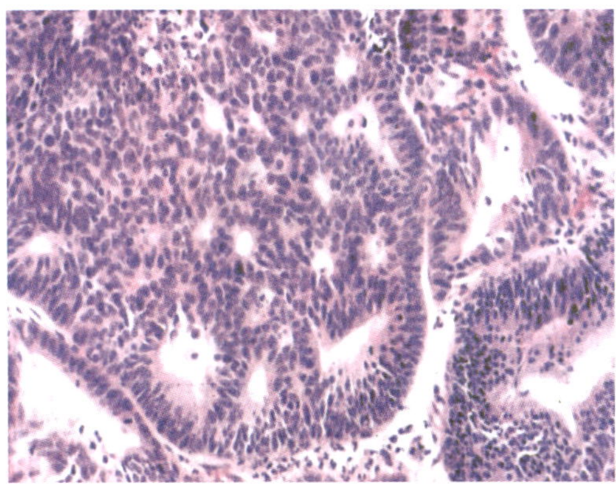

FIGURE 10.5 Microscopy of endometrial carcinoma

Spread

Spread generally occurs by invasion of myometrium and direct contiguity to the periuterine structures. Dissemination to the regional lymph nodes eventually occurs and metastasis to the lung, liver and bones will occur in the late stages of the disease.

Clinical Features

Carcinoma of the endometrium produces irregular vaginal bleeding with excessive leucorrhea. Postmenopausal bleeding is another important feature.

Prognosis

It has a very poor prognosis. Overall three years survival rate is 50 percent.

CARCINOMA OF THE CERVIX

Carcinoma of the cervix is one of the most common cancers seen in women. Cervical cancer (SCC) has been extensively studied and a direct relationship has been established ranging from squamous metaplasia, dysplasia, carcinoma *in situ* and invasive cervical cancer. Pap smear is a very useful tool in detecting the inflammatory changes and premalignant changes of dysplasia, well in advance so that it can be treated. Pap smear is taken from the transformation zone where endo- and ecto-cervix meet. The sample is taken using Ayer's spatula and smeared on the slides which are fixed in methanol, stained with Papanicolaou stain and studied. The morphology of the cells is studied and this is called as exfoliative cytology as it involves the study of cells exfoliated from the cervix.

Etiology and Pathogenesis

Extensive study into the pathogenesis of cervical cancer has shown that the causative agent is Human papilloma virus (HPV) which is a sexually transmitted agent. Specific HPV types, called the high-risk HPV are associated with the causation of cancer. These include types 16, 18, 31, 33, 35, 39, 45, 51, 52, 56, 58, 59 and 68. It is hypothesized that a molecular interaction between the virus and the host factors result in the causation of carcinoma cervix.

Risk factors associated with the development of cervical cancer are:

- Early age at first intercourse
- Multiple sexual partners
- Increased parity
- A male partner with multiple previous sexual partners
- Infection with/presence of high-risk HPV
- Other genital infections such as *Chlamydia*.

Cervical Intraepithelial Neoplasia

This refers to the precancerous condition associated with cervical cancer. These changes are classified in different ways.

Cervical Intraepithelial Neoplasia (CIN) I

These lesions usually exhibit nuclear enlargement and hyperchromasia with cytoplasmic halo, caused due to increased viral load (koilocytotic atypia). These changes are seen in the lower epithelial cells only.

Cervical Intraepithelial Neoplasia II

In this, the cells are atypical with increased nuclear-cytoplasmic ratio, variation in nuclear size, loss of polarity, increased mitotic figures and abnormal mitosis. These changes are seen in the lower one-third of the squamous epithelium.

Cervical Intraepithelial Neoplasia III (Carcinoma in situ)

Here, the atypical cells are seen in the full thickness of the squamous epithelium but does not invade the basement membrane. The morphology of cells is similar to that seen in CIN II (Fig. 10.6).

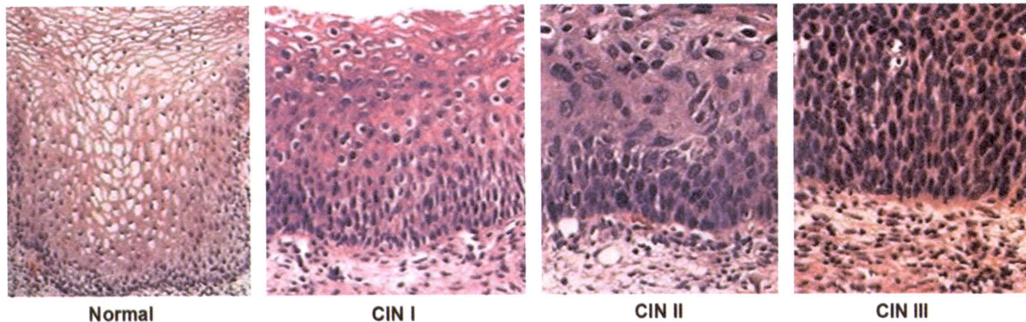

FIGURE 10.6 Microscopic picture of CIN I, II and III

Since CIN is explained with respect to the number of cells involved from the basal layer, it is difficult to quantify in the Pap smears which is exfoliative cytology. So, another classification was introduced:

a. Low grade squamous intraepithelial lesion (LSIL), which includes CIN I.
b. High grade squamous intraepithelial lesion (HSIL), which includes CIN II and CIN III.

Squamous Cell Carcinoma

The peak incidence of squamous cell carcinoma (SCC) of cervix is around 40 to 45 years.

Morphology

Gross

Invasive SCC presents in three different forms:

1. Fungating or exophytic type.
2. Ulcerating type.
3. Infiltrative type.

Microscopy

Histologically, most of the SCCs are composed of relatively large cells, either keratinizing (well differentiated) or nonkeratinizing. Few of them are poorly differentiated or small cell carcinomas (Fig. 10.7).

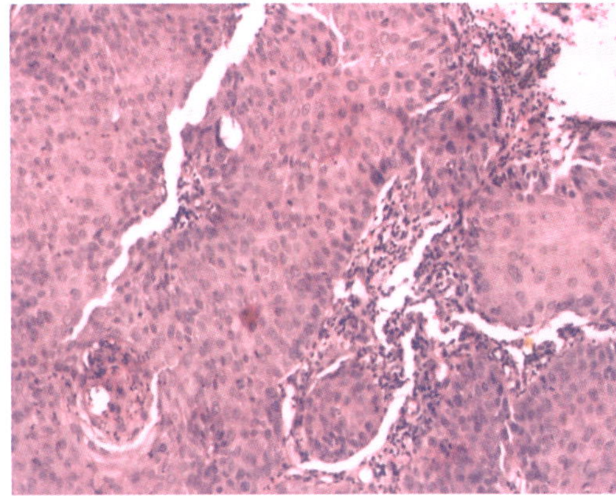

FIGURE 10.7 Microscopic picture of squamous cell carcinoma of the cervix

Clinical Features

Regular screening of all women in their reproductive age by Pap smears is highly recommended. CIN I revert back to normal on timely detection and treatment. Regular follow-up is needed for all patients with intraepithelial lesion.

The SCC spreads by involving the upper third of vaginal wall in the early stages and urinary bladder, ureter and rectal mucosa by direct extension in the later stages. With current methods of treatment, five years survival rate is at least 95 percent for early cancers. However, the prognosis worsens as the cancer becomes invasive.

ECTOPIC GESTATION

Ectopic gestation is the term applied to implantation of the fetus in any site other than the normal uterine location.

The most common site is the fallopian tubes (90%) followed by ovary and abdominal cavity. The most important predisposing conditions are pelvic inflammatory disease with chronic salpingitis, others include peritubal adhesions. Intrauterine contraceptive devices also increase the risk of ectopic pregnancy.

Morphology

In tubal pregnancy, the placenta is poorly attached to the wall of the tube. This leads to hemorrhage within the tube called as hematosalpinx. On microscopic examination, tubal fimbriae are seen along with gestational villi. These villi are lined by cytotrophoblast and syncytiotrophoblast and decidualization.

Clinical Features

Ectopic pregnancy usually presents as sudden onset. Severe abdominal pain about 6 weeks after a previous normal menstrual period, when rupture of the tube leads to pelvic hemorrhage. In such cases, the patient may rapidly go into a shock-like state and develop acute abdomen. Timely intervention and treatment is of utmost importance.

HYDATIDIFORM MOLE (VESICULAR MOLE)

Hydatidiform mole is characterized by cystic swelling of chorionic villi, accompanied by variable trophoblastic proliferation.

Clinically, these patients present in the fourth or fifth month of pregnancy with vaginal bleeding. The uterus is larger than what is expected for the duration of pregnancy.

Types of Mole

There are two types of benign, noninvasive moles: Complete mole and partial mole. The differences between the two are shown in the Table 10.1 and Figure 10.8.

TABLE 10.1 Differences between complete and partial mole

Feature	*Complete mole*	*Partial mole*
Karyotype	46, XX (46, XY)	Triploid
Villous edema	All villi	Some villi
Trophoblast proliferation	Diffuse; circumferential	Focal; slight
Atypia	Often present	Absent
Serum hCG	Elevated	Less elevated
hCG in tissue	++++	+
Behavior	2% choriocarcinoma	Rare

Morphology

Partial mole is diagnosed in early spontaneous abortions or later. Careful dissection may disclose a small, usually collapsed amniotic sac. Fetal parts are frequently seen in partial moles, but are never seen in complete moles. The complete mole classically presents with a uterine cavity filled with a delicate, friable mass. This mass consists of thin walled, translucent, cystic, grape-like structures which harbor swollen edematous (hydropic) villi (Fig. 10.9).

Microscopy

On histologic examination, partial mole demonstrates villous hydrops and architectural disturbance in only a proportion of villi. The trophoblastic proliferation is minimal and limited to the syncytiotrophoblast.

Complete moles show hydropic swelling of most chorionic villi and absence of vascularization of the villi. The villi are swollen with central cavitation called the cisterns (Fig. 10.10).

Clinical Features

Most of the patients of partial and complete moles present with spontaneous abortion or

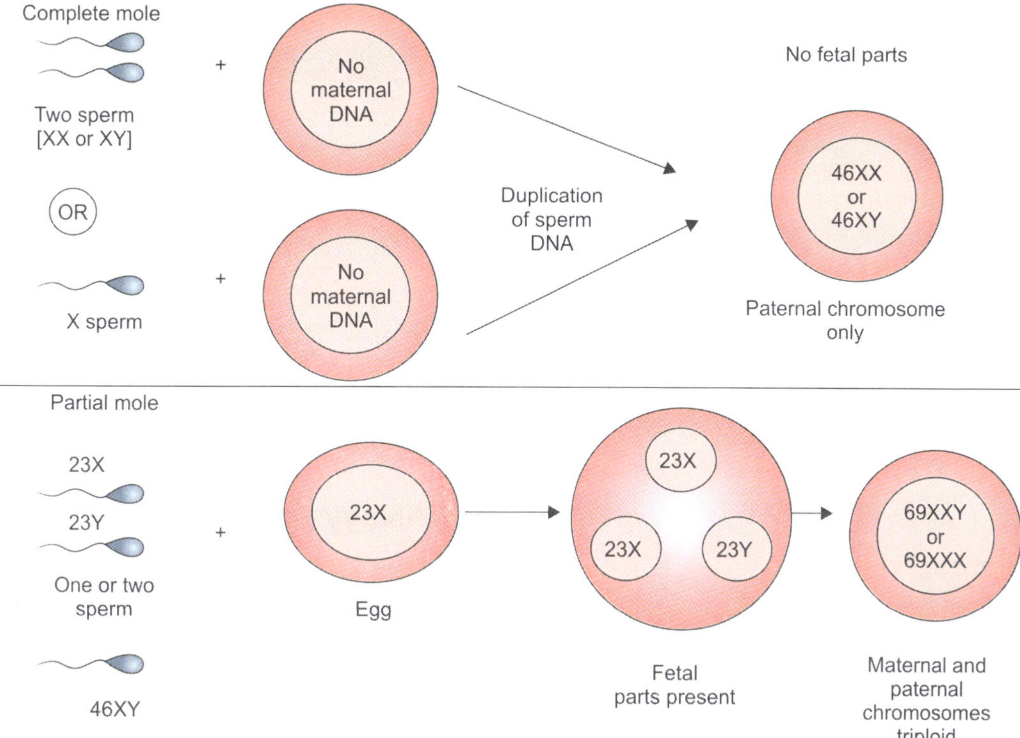

FIGURE 10.8 Diagrammatic representation of patterns of fertilization seen in complete and partial mole

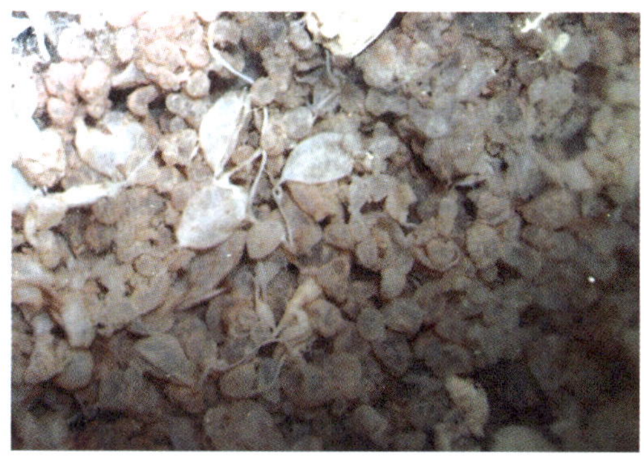

FIGURE 10.9 Gross picture of hydatidiform mole

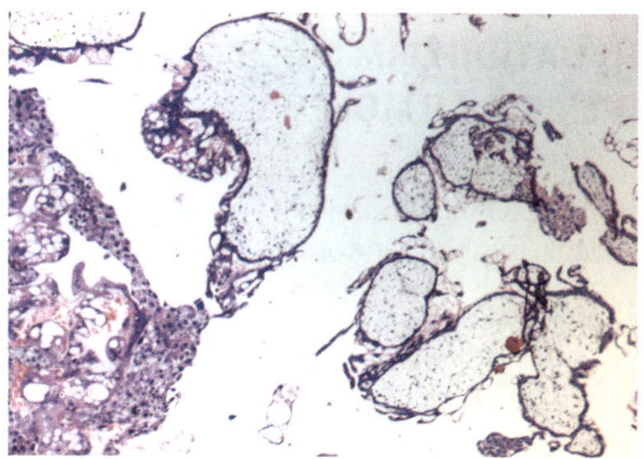

FIGURE 10.10 Microscopy of hydatidiform mole

undergo curettage due to abnormalities in ultrasound. Watery fluid and bits of small, grape-like masses can be seen in the uterine contents. Thorough curettage of the uterine cavity and serial estimation of human chorionic gonadotropin (hCG) levels is the treatment of choice. Partial mole does not progress to malignancy. Only two percent of complete moles will progress to develop choriocarcinoma.

CHORIOCARCINOMA

Gestational choriocarcinoma is an epithelial malignant neoplasm of trophoblastic cells, derived from any form of previously normal or abnormal pregnancy. Choriocarcinoma is a rapidly invasive, widely metastasizing malignant neoplasm, but if once identified, it responds well to chemotherapy. Fifty percent of the cases arise in hydatidiform mole, 25 percent in previous abortions and 22 percent in normal pregnancies. Three percent arises in ectopic pregnancy.

Morphology

Gross

Classically, choriocarcinoma is soft, fleshy, yellow-white tumor. It shows large pale areas of ischemic necrosis, foci of cystic softening and extensive hemorrhage.

Microscopy

It is an epithelial tumor that does not produce chorionic villi. It grows by abnormal proliferation of cytotrophoblast and syncytiotrophoblast. The tumor invades the underlying myometrium, frequently penetrates the lymphatics and blood vessels. In some cases, it can metastasize to the lungs, brain, bone marrow and other organs (Fig. 10.11).

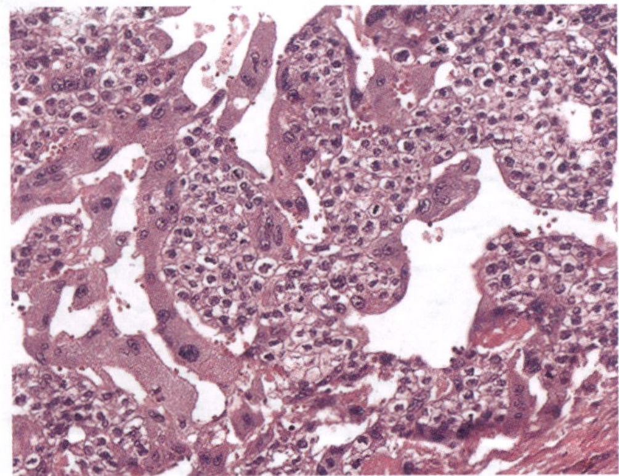

FIGURE 10.11 Microscopy of choriocarcinoma

Clinical Features

Uterine choriocarcinoma presents with symptoms of irregular spotting of a brown, bloody, sometimes foul smelling fluid. This discharge may appear in the course of an apparently normal pregnancy, miscarriage, or after curettage. The titers of hCG are elevated more than that seen in hydatidiform mole. Widespread metastasis is common in this tumor. Favored sites of involvement are the lungs (50%) and vagina (30–40%).

Treatment depends on the type and stage of the tumor. It usually responds well to a combination of surgery and chemotherapy. A 100 percent cure or remission has been achieved in the treatment of this disease.

OVARIAN TUMORS

Tumors of the ovary are common forms of neoplasia of female genital tract. There are numerous types of ovarian tumors, both benign and malignant. About 80 percent are benign, occurring commonly in young women between 20 and 45 years. The malignant tumors are more common in older women between 40 and 65 years.

Classification

The tumors of the ovary have been classified by the World Health Organization and are given in Table 10.2.

Only few tumors of the ovary are described in this book. For the detailed discussion of ovarian neoplasms, the reader is referred to other books.

Risk Factors for the Development of Ovarian Tumors

In general, the risk factors for ovarian tumors are less clear than other genital neoplasms. Nulliparity, family history and genetic mutations play a role in the development of ovarian tumors. There is a higher frequency in for the development of ovarian tumors unmarried women and in women with low parity.

TABLE 10.2 WHO classification of ovarian neoplasms

Surface Epithelial Stromal Tumors
Serous tumors
- Benign (Cystadenoma)
- Cystadenoma of borderline malignancy
- Malignant (serous cystadenocarcinoma)

Mucinous tumors
- Benign
- Of borderline malignancy
- Malignant

Endometrioid tumors
- Benign
- Of borderline malignancy
- Malignant

Epithelial—stromal
- Adenosarcoma
- Mixed mesodermal müllerian tumor

Clear cell tumors
- Benign
- Of borderline malignancy
- Malignant

Transitional cell tumors
- Brenner tumor
- Brenner tumor of borderline malignancy
- Malignant Brenner tumor
- Transitional cell carcinoma (Non-Brenner type)

Sex Cord—Stromal Tumors
Granulosa—Stromal cell tumors
- Granulosa cell tumor
- Tumors of the thecoma—fibroma group

Sertoli—stromal cell tumors; androblastoma
Sex cord tumor with annular tubules
Gynandroblastoma
Steroid (lipid) cell tumor

Germ Cell Tumors
Teratoma
- Immature
- Mature (adult)
  - Solid
  - Cystic (Dermoid cyst)
  - Monodermal

Example: Struma ovarii, carcinoid

Dysgerminoma
Yolk sac tumor
Mixed germ cell tumor

Malignant, Not Otherwise Specified
Metastatic Non-ovarian Cancer

SEROUS TUMORS

These neoplasms are common and mostly cystic. The cyst wall is lined by tall columnar, ciliated epithelial cells and is filled with clear serous fluid. About 75 percent are benign or of borderline malignancy, and 25 percent are malignant. The age of occurrence is between 20 and 50 years.

Morphology

Gross

Serous cystadenoma is the benign cystic tumor with smooth glistening cyst wall.

Borderline serous tumors present with increased number of papillary projections into the cyst wall.

Malignant serous cystadenocarcinomas present with more irregular solid areas with fixation or nodularity of the capsule.

Microscopy

Serous cystadenomas which are benign are lined by single layer of ciliated columnar epithelium (Fig. 10.12).

Borderline serous tumors present with stromal papillae with stratification of the epithelium and mild atypia of the cells.

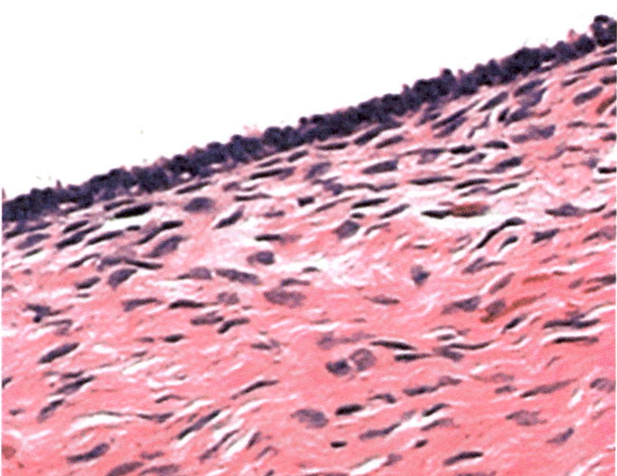

FIGURE 10.12 Microscopy of serous cystadenoma

Cystadenocarcinomas exhibit even more complex growth pattern, with infiltration of the underlying stroma by the tumor cells. Individual tumor cells show hyperchromatic nucleus, prominent nucleolus and abnormal mitosis. Concentric calcifications called psammoma bodies are characteristically seen in this tumor (Fig. 10.13).

MUCINOUS TUMORS

These tumors are less common than the serous tumors accounting for about 25 percent of all ovarian tumors. They occur principally in the middle adult life.

Morphology

Gross

Mucinous tumors contain multiple cysts of varying sizes. They are thus multiloculated and are filled with sticky, gelatinous fluid rich in glycoproteins.

Microscopy

Benign mucinous tumors are lined by tall columnar epithelial cells with apical mucin and no cilia (Fig. 10.14).

Mucinous tumors of borderline malignancy exhibit stratification, papillary or gland-alike architecture and mild nuclear atypia.

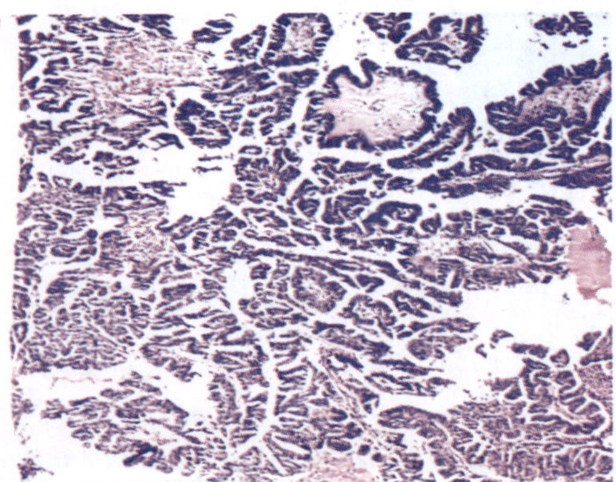

FIGURE 10.13 Microscopy of serous cystadenocarcinoma

Mucinous cystadenocarcinomas contain solid growth pattern with epithelial cell atypia, stratification, loss of glandular architecture and necrosis. These tumors are invasive (Fig. 10.15).

Pseudomyxoma peritonei is a condition, which consists of ovarian tumor with extensive mucinous ascites, cystic epithelial implants on peritoneal surface and adhesions.

GERM CELL TUMORS

Germ cell tumors constitue 15 to 20 percent of all ovarian neoplasms. Most common is benign cystic teratoma.

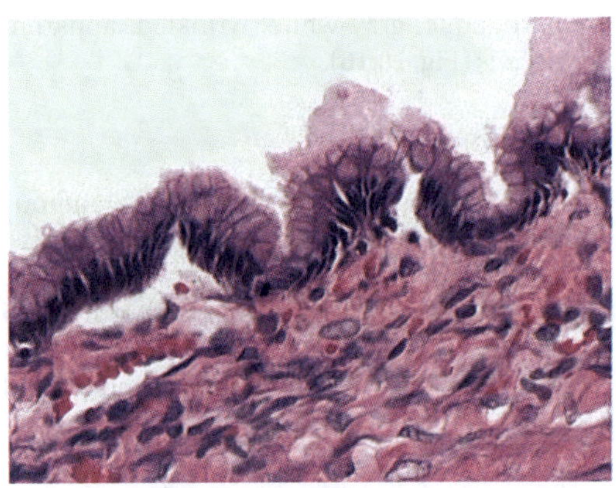

FIGURE 10.14 Microscopy of mucinous cystadenoma

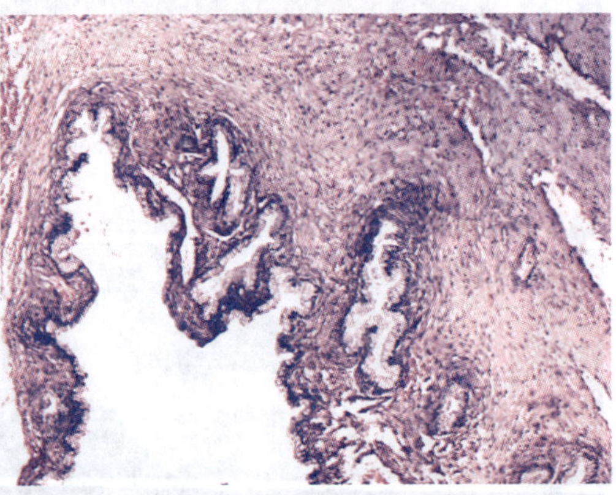

FIGURE 10.15 Microscopic picture of mucinous cystadenocarcinoma

TERATOMA

Teratomas are divided into:

1. Mature (Benign cystic teratoma)
2. Immature (malignant)
3. Monodermal or highly specialized

Benign cystic teratomas are also known as dermoid cysts.

Morphology

Gross

Benign tumors are bilateral in 10 percent of cases. Grossly, they are uniloculated cysts containing hair, tooth and cheesy sebaceous material. Cut section shows a thin wall cyst lined by an opaque, gray-white, wrinkled, apparent epidermis (Fig. 10.16).

Microscopy

The cyst wall is lined by stratified squamous epithelium with underlying sebaceous glands, hair shafts and other skin adnexal structures. Many times, structures derived from other two germ layers such as cartilage, bone, thyroid tissue and other organs can be identified (Fig. 10.17).

Immature malignant teratomas contain structures which are very immature and resemble that seen in the fetus or the embryo. Grossly, these tumors are more solid with areas of hemorrhage and necrosis. Histologically, many immature structures like immature cartilage and neuroepithelial tissue is seen. This tumor grows rapidly and frequently penetrates the capsule with local spread and metastasis.

BREAST

The mammary gland in the females rests between the second and the sixth ribs on the pectoralis major muscle.

Breast Tumors

Fibroadenoma

Fibroadenoma is the most common benign tumor of the female breast. It arises from the intralobular stroma of the breast. Most patients are between 15 and 30 years of age.

Pathology

Gross: It is usually a small, well encapsulated, solitary or multiple, spherical mass. Cut surface

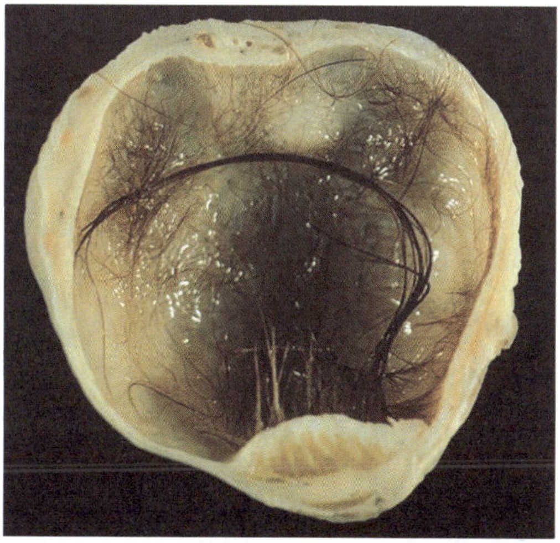

FIGURE 10.16 Gross picture of mature cystic teratoma

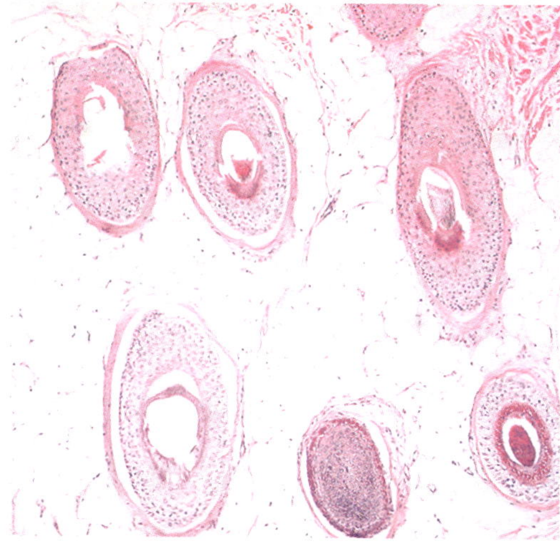

FIGURE 10.17 Microscopy of mature cystic teratoma

is gray-white, myxoid and shows slit-like spaces formed by compressed ducts.

Microscopy: The proliferating stroma compresses the ducts so that, they are reduced to slit like clefts lined by ductal epithelium. The stroma sometimes is myxomatous (Fig. 10.18).

Clinical Features

It presents as a lump in the breast which can be single or multiple, unilateral or bilateral, freely mobile.

Treatment is excision. Malignant transformation is very rare.

CARCINOMA OF BREAST

Carcinoma of breast is among the most common of cancers in women.

Etiopathogenesis

Large numbers of risk factors have been identified.

- Genetic factors
  - Family history—first degree relatives of women with breast cancer have two to six fold higher risk.
  - Mutations in BRCA1 gene located in chromosome 17 and *BRCA2* gene on chromosome 13.
- Hormonal factors—estrogen excess
- Environmental and dietary factors—consumption of large amounts of animal fats, high calorie food, cigarette smoking and alcohol.
- Pre-existing breast lesions like atypical ductal hyperplasia.

Carcinoma breast arises from ductal epithelium in 90 percent of the cases and while other 10 percent arises from lobular epithelium.

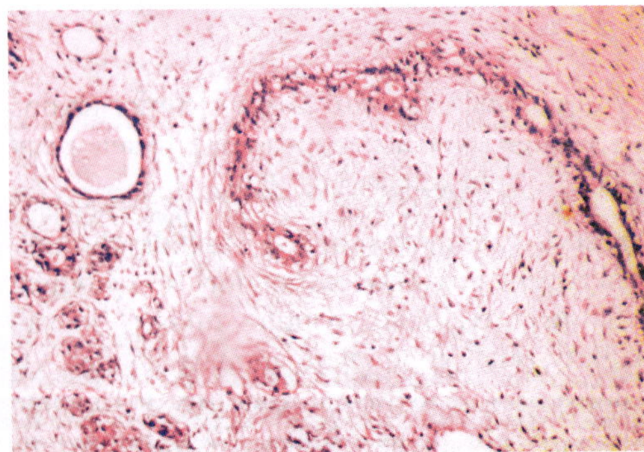

FIGURE 10.18 Microscopy of fibroadenoma breast

Classification

- Noninvasive (*in situ*) carcinoma
  - Intraductal carcinoma
  - Lobular carcinoma *in situ*
- Invasive carcinoma
  - Infiltrating (invasive) ductal carcinoma— NOS (not otherwise specified)
  - Infiltrating (invasive) lobular carcinoma
  - Medullary carcinoma
  - Colloid (mucinous) carcinoma
  - Papillary carcinoma
  - Tubular carcinoma
  - Adenoid cystic carcinoma
  - Secretory carcinoma
  - Inflammatory carcinoma
  - Carcinoma with metaplasia
- Paget's disease of the nipple.

Invasive Carcinoma

Infiltrating Ductal Carcinoma—NOS

Gross: The tumor is irregular, hard and cuts with a grating sound. Cut surface shows grey white chalky streaks (Fig. 10.19).

Microscopy: Anaplastic tumor cells form solid nests, cords, and poorly formed glandular structures. These tumor cells infiltrate into the stroma and also into lymphatic and perineural spaces. The stroma is usually desmoplastic (Fig. 10.20).

Medullary Carcinoma

Gross: It is usually a large, well circumscribed, rounded mass that is soft and fleshy.

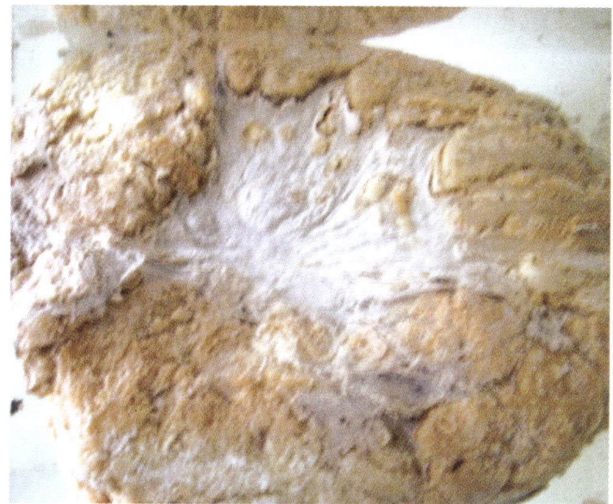

FIGURE 10.19 Gross picture of invasive ductal carcinoma breast

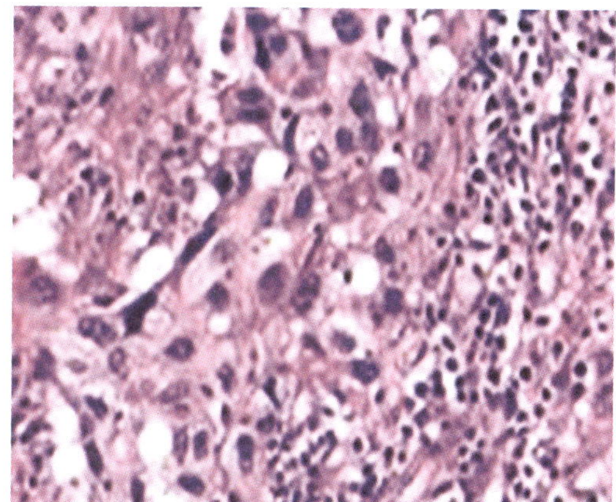

FIGURE 10.21 Microscopy of medullary carcinoma breast

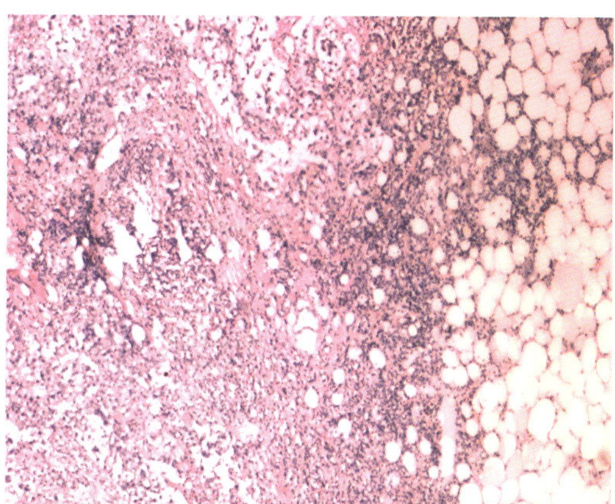

FIGURE 10.20 Microscopy of invasive ductal carcinoma breast

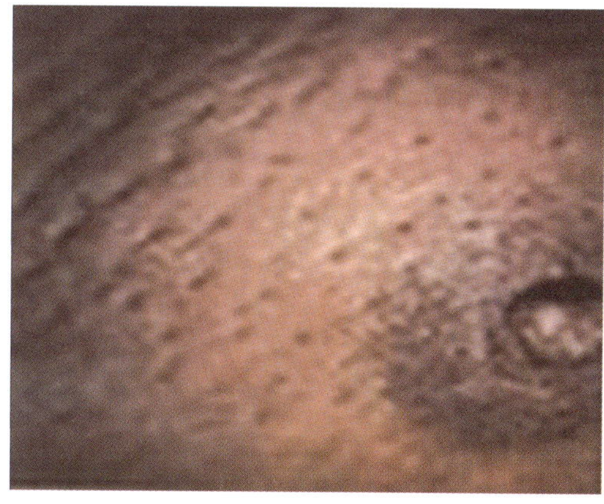

FIGURE 10.22 Peau d'orange appearance of breast

Microscopy: Sheets of large, pleomorphic cells with abundant cytoplasm, vesicular nucleus and atypical mitotic figures. These cells have a pushing margin. Stroma is scanty and has a prominent lymphoplasmacytic infiltrate (Fig. 10.21).

Clinical features: It presents as a solitary, painless, palpable lump. There may be bleeding per nipple and retracted nipple. In the later stages, due to obstruction of the lymphatics by tumor cells, the skin over the tumor attains an orange peel like appearance called *peau d'orange* appearance (Fig. 10.22).

Spread: Carcinoma breast spreads through lymphatic channels, commonly to produce enlarged regional lymph nodes mostly axillary and internal mammary nodes. It may also spread hematogenously to involve the opposite breast, lungs, liver, bone and brain.

Emphasis is on the early diagnosis by various methods.

They are:

- Clinical examination
- Mammography
- Xeroradiography and thermography
- Fine needle aspiration cytology (FNAC)
- Intraoperative imprint cytology
- Stereotactic biopsy
- Frozen section
- Excision biopsy.

Staging of Breast Carcinoma—AJCC Staging

Stage Tis-*in situ* carcinoma

- Tumor < 2 cm in diameter
  - No nodal spread
- Tumor > 2 cm in diameter
  - Regional lymph nodes enlarged
- Tumor ≤ 5 cm in diameter
  - Regional lymph nodes involved on same side
- Tumor ≥ 5 cm in diameter
  - Supraclavicular and infraclavicular lymph nodes involved
- Tumor of any size
  - With or without regional spread but with distant metastasis.

Prognostic Markers for Invasive Carcinoma Breast

- Tumor size
- Lymph node involvement
- Histologic grading
- Histologic type
- Mitosis
- Estrogen-progesterone receptors
- Proliferation markers
- Dysregulation of oncogene
- Vascular factors.

CHAPTER 11

Central Nervous System

NORMAL STRUCTURE

The central nervous system (CNS) consists of brain and spinal cord encased in skull and vertebrae. The weight of the brain in males is about 1400 g and 1250 g in females. Brain is divided into cerebrum, cerebellum, pons and medulla. The main cells of the CNS are neurons, glia and the cells that compose meninges and blood vessels. The brain is covered by a tough fibrous sheath called dura mater and leptomeninges which includes pia mater and arachnoid mater (Fig. 11.1).

Histologically the two main components are the neurons and neuroglia. The neurons are specialized cells involved in conduction of impulses. The neuroglia support the neurons and they are astrocytes, oligodendrocytes and ependymal cells.

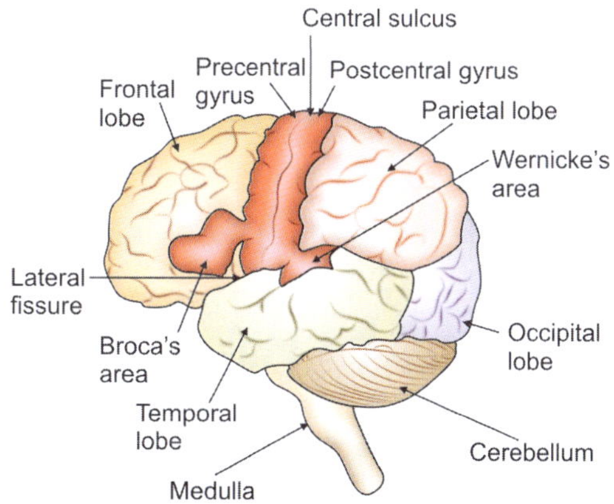

FIGURE 11.1 Diagrammatic representation of anatomy of central nervous system

The common disorders of CNS are:

- Developmental anomalies
- Hydrocephalus
- Infections like meningitis and encephalitis
- Cerebrovascular diseases
- Trauma causing epidural and subdural hematomas
- Demyelinating diseases
- Tumors of the CNS.

HYDROCEPHALUS

Increased volume of CSF within the skull, along with dilatation of the ventricles is called hydrocephalus.

Classification

Hydrocephalus is classified into primary and secondary hydrocephalus.

Primary Hydrocephalus

It is defined as increase in the volume of CSF along with increase in the intracranial pressure. It is more common than secondary hydrocephalus.

Causes
- Obstruction to the flow of CSF—most common and also called obstructive hydrocephalus
- Overproduction of CSF
- Deficient reabsorption of CSF.

Hydrocephalus is further divided into communicating and noncommunicating hydrocephalus depending on the site of obstruction.

In communicating hydrocephalus, the obstruction is in the subarachnoid space. It results in the enlargement of the ventricular system but the CSF flows freely between the dilated ventricles and the spinal canal. The causes are nonobstructive which are overproduction of CSF and deficient reabsorption.

In noncommunicating hydrocephalus, the site of obstruction is in the third ventricle or the exit of fourth ventricle. Here there is enlargement of ventricles, but the CSF cannot pass into the subarachnoid space. The causes are congenital and acquired. The congenital causes are stenosis of aqueduct, Arnold-Chiari malformation and Dandy-Walker malformation the acquired causes being tumors, inflammatory lesions and hemorrhage.

Secondary Hydrocephalus

It is less common and is characterized by compensatory increase of CSF due to loss of neural tissue without any elevation in the intracranial pressure. The causes are cerebral atrophy and infarction.

Morphology
- *Gross*: Dilated ventricles with thinning and stretching of the brain can be seen.
- *Microscopy*: Periventricular interstitial edema and damaged ependymal lining.

Clinical Features

In congenital hydrocephalus, the head circumference of the newborn increases rapidly. The fontanelles bulge out as the skull bones have not yet fused.

In acquired hydrocephalus, symptoms of increased intracranial pressure like headache, nausea, vomiting and papilledema can be seen.

Treatment of hydrocephalus is usually surgical.

MENINGITIS

Meningitis is the inflammation of meninges, either due to injury or infection.

When it is involves the dura mater, it is called pachymeningitis. When pia-arachnoid is involved, it is leptomeningitis. It is mostly due to infection. Chemical meningitis and carcinomatous meningitis are the other types.

Infectious meningitis is broadly classified into three:
1. Acute pyogenic (bacterial) meningitis
2. Acute lymphocytic (viral or aseptic) meningitis
3. Chronic meningitis (tuberculosis or *Cryptococcus*).

Acute Pyogenic Meningitis

It is acute infection of the pia-arachnoid and of the CSF enclosed in the subarachnoid space.

Etiopathogenesis

- *In neonates: Escherichia coli*, Group B streptococci.
- *In infants and children: Haemophilus influenzae, Neisseria meningitidis.*
- *In adults: Streptococcus pneumoniae, Neisseria meningitidis*, mycobacteria.

Pathology

Gross: CSF becomes turbid or purulent.

Microscopy: Neutrophils are seen in the subarachnoid space and in the meninges.

Clinical Features

The common features are severe headache, fever, drowsiness, vomiting, coma and occasionally convulsions.

Signs

Nuchal rigidity (neck stiffness) is an important sign. The triad of signs are nuchal rigidity, high

fever and altered sensorium. Other signs are photophobia, irritability and delirium.

Laboratory Diagnosis

The diagnosis is confirmed by CSF examination. CSF is aspirated through lumbar puncture and is tested for cells, protein and glucose. The type of WBCs seen predominantly gives us a clue as to whether it is bacterial or viral infection. Gram staining of the sample may demonstrate bacteria. In bacterial meningitis, the CSF appears cloudy with elevated pressure of more than 180 mm water. Neutrophils are increased up to 100,000/μL. CSF protein is raised to more than 50 mg/dL and sugar is decreased to less than 40 mg/dL.

Acute Lymphocytic (Viral or Aseptic) Meningitis

Acute viral meningitis is common in children and young adults. The causative viruses are mumps, enteroviruses, coxsackie virus, Epstein-Barr virus, ECHO viruses and herpes simplex II.

Pathology

Gross: There might not be any distinctive change.

Microscopy: Lymphocytes may be seen in the meninges.

Clinical Features

The symptoms are same as that of bacterial meningitis but are mild and of short duration and is self-limiting.

Laboratory Diagnosis

The CSF in viral meningitis is either clear or turbid. The CSF pressure is increased to more than 250 mm water. Lymphocytes are increased up to 100 cells/μL. CSF protein is usually normal or slightly reduced. CSF sugar is usually normal and CSF is bacteriologically sterile.

Chronic Meningitis

It can either be due to bacteria (tuberculous meningitis) or fungus (cryptococcal meningitis).

Tuberculous meningitis may occur due to hematogenous spread from the infection elsewhere in the body. Cryptococcal meningitis is most commonly seen in immunocompromised patients.

Pathology

Gross: Subarachnoid space shows thick exudate in tuberculous meningitis. Tubercles of 1-2 mm in diameter can also be seen. In cryptococcal meningitis, the exudates are gelatinous and translucent.

Microscopy: In tuberculous meningitis, granulomas with or without caseation necrosis and giant cells can be seen. In later stages, fibrous adhesions develop causing hydrocephalus. Zn stain can demonstrate the bacilli.

Chronic inflammatory cells like lymphocytes and plasma cells are seen in cryptococcal meningitis. Abundant capsulated cryptococci can be demonstrated.

Clinical Features

Headache, vomiting, malaise are the clinical symptoms in tuberculous meningitis. Cryptococcal meningitis may be fatal.

Laboratory Diagnosis

Cerebrospinal fluid (CSF) is either clear or turbid. It forms a fibrin web when left standing. The pressure is increased to more than 300 mm water. The cells seen are lymphocytes and macrophages with raised protein and decreased glucose. Ziehl-Neelsen staining of the centrifuged deposit of CSF shows tubercle bacilli. Cryptococci can be demonstrated by India ink preparation of CSF (Table 11.1).

ENCEPHALITIS

Encephalitis is the infection of the brain parenchyma. It is due to bacterial, viral, fungal

TABLE 11.1 CSF findings in various types of meningitis

Type	*CSF pressure*	*Cells*	*Proteins*	*Glucose*
Normal	60–150 mm water	0–4 lymphocytes/ μL	15–45 mg/dL	50–80 mg/dL
Acute bacterial meningitis	>180 mm water	1000–100,000 neutrophils/μL	Markedly increased	Decreased
Acute lymphocytic meningitis	>250 mm water	10–100 mononuclear cells /μL	Increased	Normal
Chronic meningitis	>300 mm water	100–1000 mononuclear cells/μL	Increased	Decreased

and protozoal infections. Bacterial infection of the brain can cause brain abscess which are localized suppuration of the brain, tuberculoma, an intracranial mass secondary to tuberculosis of brain and neurosyphilis seen in the tertiary stage of syphilis.

The most common viral agents causing infection of the brain are HIV, herpes zoster virus, cytomegalovirus, rabies virus and poliovirus. The common fungal organisms include cryptococci, *Aspergillus, Histoplasma,* mucor, *Candida, Blastomyces* and other fungi.

Pathology

Gross

Brain abscess grossly appears as a localized area of necrosis and edema. Tuberculoma is seen as a central area of caseation necrosis surrounded by fibrous capsule.

Microscopy

Brain abscess show liquefactive necrosis surrounded by edema, zone of gliosis and acute inflammatory cells. The meninges and CSF are also involved. In tuberculoma, there is central caseation necrosis surrounded by granulomatous reaction. Calcification can also be seen sometimes.

In viral encephalitis, chronic inflammatory cells can be seen in the perivascular area along with clusters of microglial cells and intranuclear inclusion bodies. The characteristic Negri bodies can be seen as intracytoplasmic inclusions in rabies virus infection.

Clinical Features

Patients suffer from fever, headache, weakness, seizures, vomiting and focal neurological deficits depending on the location of the lesion. Less commonly, stiffness of the neck and limbs, irritability and anorexia can be seen.

Laboratory Diagnosis

Cerebrospinal fluid (CSF) is examined which shows increased protein and leucocytes with normal glucose. Diagnosis is made by detection of specific antibodies against a specific viral agent.

CEREBROVASCULAR DISEASES

One or more blood vessels of the brain are in volved in these diseases. Thrombosis, embolism, atherosclerosis, arteritis, aneurysm, trauma, hy pertensive arteriosclerosis and developmental malformations are the various pathological processes. Thromboembolic infarction (80%), cerebral and cerebellar hemorrhage (10%) and subarachnoid hemorrhage (about 5%) are the major cerebrovascular problems.

There are two main forms of cerebrovascular diseases. They are:

1. Diseases due to ischemic brain damage
2. Diseases due to intracranial hemorrhage.

The characteristic clinical feature of the cerebrovascular disease is stroke syndrome, which is sudden onset of focal neurological deficit manifesting as hemiplegia and coma.

Risk Factors

The important risk factors are old age, hypertension, diabetes and cigarette smoking. Other risks include alcohol, hypercholesterolemia and genetics.

Ischemic Brain Damage

There are two patterns of ischemic brain damage:

1. Hypoxic-ischemic encephalopathy due to generalized cerebral hypoperfusion.
2. Cerebral infarction due to localized cessation of blood supply.

In conditions like shock where there is significant fall of systemic arterial blood pressure, there is fall in the cerebral perfusion resulting in hypoxic-ischemic encephalopathy.

In cerebral infarction, blood supply to part of the brain is decreased causing necrosis of the brain tissue. This is due to hypoxia which can be induced by arterial occlusion either due to thrombosis or embolism, venous occlusion, nonocclusive causes like compression of arteries.

Pathology

Gross

In hypoxic-ischemic encephalopathy, there is focal softening. In cerebral infarction, infarcts may be anemic or hemorrhagic. Anemic infarct is soft and swollen with a blurring junction between grey and white matter. A hemorrhagic infarct is red.

Microscopy

In hypoxic-ischemic encephalopathy, there is death of the neurons and are replaced by fibrillary gliosis. In cerebral infarction, the infracted area is infiltrated by neutrophils. After 2–3 days, there is invasion of macrophages and astrocytes along with vascular proliferation. After 3–4 months, cystic infarcts are formed which are called lacunar infarcts.

Intracranial Hemorrhage

There are three types of intracranial hemorrhage—intracerebral, subarachnoid, subdural and extradural.

Intracerebral Hemorrhage

The most common causes of intracerebral hemorrhage are hypertension, rupture of aneurysms, arteriovenous malformations and trauma.

The common sites of hypertensive intracerebral hemorrhage are the region of basal ganglia, pons and the cerebellar cortex.

Clinical Features

There is headache and rapid reduction of consciousness with signs of brainstem origin (e.g. nystagmus, ocular palsies). Gaze deviates towards the hemorrhage. Cerebellar hemorrhage sometimes causes acute hydrocephalus. Emergency surgical clot evacuation is often necessary after imaging.

Subarachnoid Hemorrhage

It means spontaneous arterial bleeding into the subarachnoid space. Subarachnoid hemorrhage (SAH) accounts for some 5 percent of strokes. It is most commonly due to rupture of aneurysm. Berry aneurysms are the most common and important. Berry aneurysms develop due to defect in the arterial media of the arterial wall at the bifurcation of arteries. They are saccular in appearance, varying in size from 1 to 2 cm or more.

The other intracranial aneurysms are mycotic and fusiform.

In most of the cases, subarachnoid hemorrhage is due to rupture of a berry aneurysm on or near the circle of Willis (Fig. 11.2).

Clinical Features of SAH

There is a sudden headache, often occipital. This is usually followed by vomiting and often by coma. The patient remains comatose or drowsy for several hours to several days. After

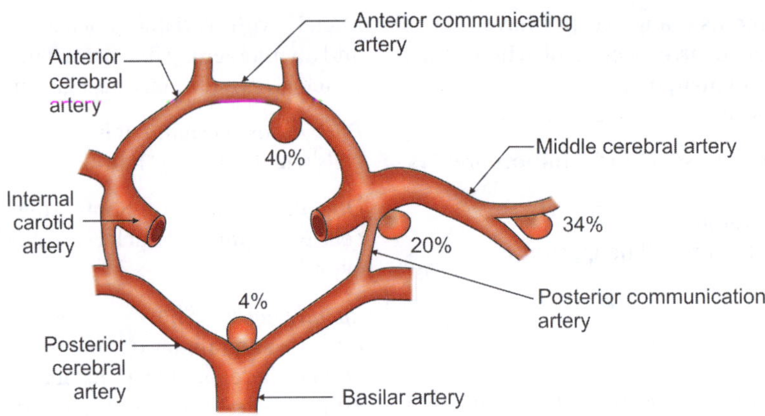

FIGURE 11.2 Diagrammatic representation of circle of Willis with aneurysms

major SAH there is neck stiffness and a positive Kernig's sign. Papilledema is sometimes present and accompanied by retinal and subhyaloid hemorrhage (tracking beneath the retinal hyaloid membrane). Minor bleeds cause few signs, but almost invariably headache. Blood in the subarachnoid space can lead to obstruction of CSF flow and hydrocephalus.

Subdural Hematoma

The subdural hematoma (SDH) means accumulation of blood in the subdural space following rupture of a vein. It usually follows a head injury, which may be trivial. The interval between injury and symptoms may be days, weeks or months. Chronic, unsuspected or spontaneous SDH is common in the elderly and in alcohol abuse.

Headache, drowsiness and confusion are common. Focal deficits such as hemiparesis or sensory loss develop. Epilepsy occasionally occurs. Stupor and coma may follow, but there is a tendency for SDH to resolve spontaneously.

Extradural Hemorrhage

This follows a linear skull vault fracture tearing a branch of the middle meningeal artery. Blood accumulates rapidly over minutes/hours in the extradural space. The most characteristic picture is of a head injury with a brief duration of unconsciousness followed by a lucid interval of recovery. The patient then develops a progressive hemiparesis and stupor, with first an ipsilateral dilated pupil, followed by bilateral fixed dilated pupils, tetraplegia and respiratory arrest.

Hemiplegia: Hemiplegia is a condition where there is paralysis of one half of the body. It is usually the result of a stroke.

Paraplegia: Paraplegia is an impairment in motor and/or sensory function of the lower extremities. It is most commonly due to spinal cord injury or a congenital condition called spina bifida.

Quadriplegia (tetraplegia): It is paralysis of all four limbs caused by damage to brain or spinal cord at a higher level. It need not necessarily be a total loss of function. Severity depends on both the level at which the spinal cord is damaged and the extent of the injury.

TUMORS OF THE CNS

Tumors of the CNS have certain unique features.

- It is sometimes difficult to differentiate between a benign and a malignant tumor causing clinical deficits and poor prognosis.
- These tumors usually cause pressure effects due to limited space in the bony

compartments and can have lethal consequences irrespective of whether it is benign or malignant.
- They rarely metastasize outside the CNS.

The four major classes of brain tumors are:
1. Gliomas
2. Neuronal tumors
3. Poorly differentiated neoplasms
4. Meningiomas.

Gliomas

Gliomas include astrocytomas, oligodendrogliomas and ependymomas and are derived from glial cells.
- *Astrocytomas*: From astrocytes
- *Oligodendrogliomas*: From oligodendrocytes
- *Ependymomas*: From ependymal cells.

Astrocytomas are further categorized into fibrillary astrocytoma, glioblastoma, pilocytic astrocytoma and pleomorphic xanthoastrocytoma depending on the histological features, distribution with in the brain, age and clinical course.

Pathology

Gross

Astrocytoma: Fibrillary astrocytoma presents as a poorly defined, gray, infiltrative tumor. Pilocytic astrocytoma is often cystic. Pleomorphic xanthoastrocytoma is common in the temporal lobe and quite superficial.

Oligodendrogliomas: These are well-circumscribed, gelatinous, gray masses with cysts, hemorrhage and calcification.

Ependymomas: In the first two decades, it is common near the fourth ventricle. In adults, spinal cord is the common location. Grossly, in the fourth ventricle, the tumors are typically solid or papillary masses extending from the floor of the ventricle.

Microscopy: Well-differentiated fibrillary astrocytoma shows increase in the glial cell nuclei, with variable nuclear pleomorphism and an intervening fine astrocytic cell processes which gives a fibrillary background (Fig. 11.3).

Pilocytic astrocytoma: It is composed of bipolar cells with long, thin "hairlike" processes.

Oligodendrogliomas: Show sheets of regular cells with spherical nuclei surrounded by a clear cytoplasm.

Ependymomas: Show cells with round to oval nuclei with granular chromatin. Between these nuclei there is dense fibrillary background. Tumor cells form gland like structures called rosettes (Fig. 11.4).

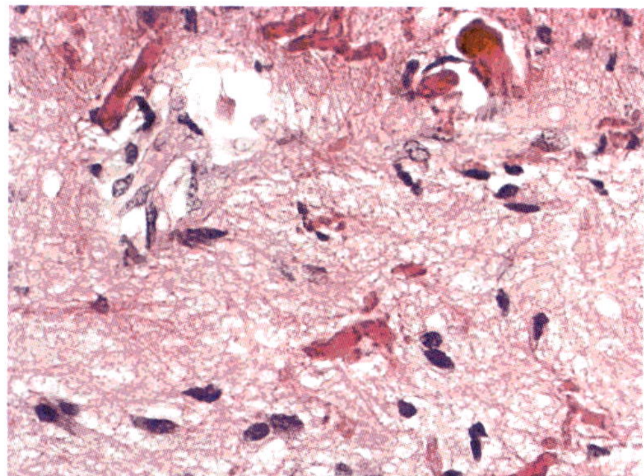

FIGURE 11.3 Microscopy of fibrillary astrocytoma

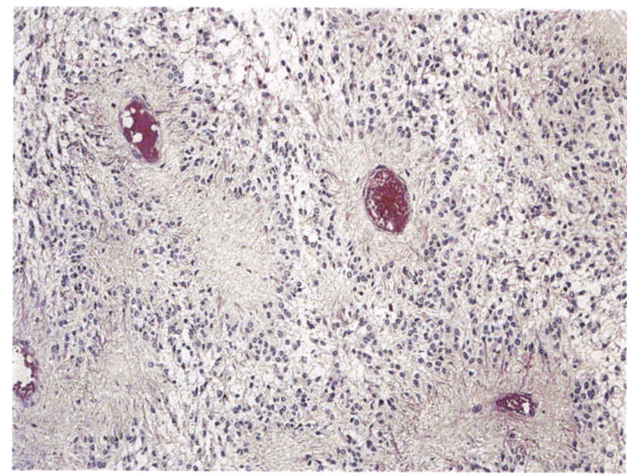

FIGURE 11.4 Microscopy of ependymoma

Clinical Features

It depends upon which part of the CNS is involved. They can cause headache, nausea, vomiting, seizures and cranial nerve disorders due to increased intracranial pressure. Optic nerve involvement can cause visual loss. Weakness and numbness in the extremities are seen when spinal cord is involved.

Treatment

It is usually by surgery, radiotherapy and chemotherapy.

Meningiomas

They are benign tumors predominantly. The cell of origin is the meningothelial cell of the arachnoid. They are seen either on the external surfaces of the brain or within the ventricular system. They are common between 20 and 60 years of age and have a slight female preponderance.

Pathology

Gross: It presents as a well-circumscribed, usually encapsulated mass with a well-defined dural base that compress the underlying brain. It spreads like a sheet on the surface of the dura sometimes and is then called en plaque variant. Extension into the overlying bone may be present.

Microscopy: The cells are uniform and are arranged in whorled clusters with numerous psammoma bodies which are nothing but lamellated calcific concretions (Fig. 11.5).

Clinical features: They present either with vague nonlocalizing symptoms or symptoms due to compression of brain.

Treatment: It is usually surgical resection.

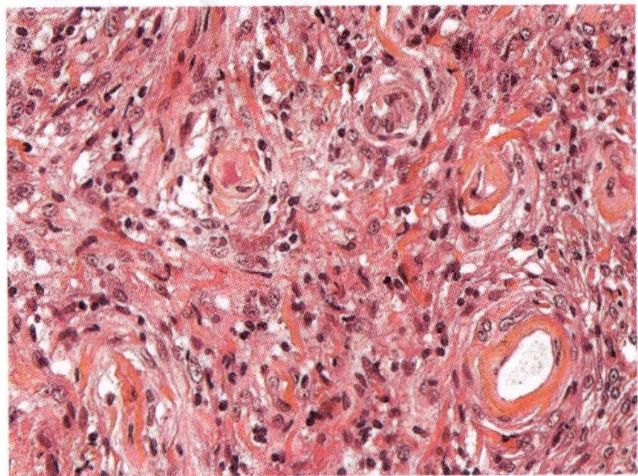

FIGURE 11.5 Microscopy of meningioma. Note the whirling pattern

Metastatic Tumors

The common primary sites from which the metastasis occurs to brain are lung, breast, skin, kidney and gastrointestinal tract.

Gross

They form sharply demarcated masses usually at the gray matter-white matter junction.

Microscopy

The tumor and the brain parenchyma is well defined except in melanoma. It has the same appearance as that of the primary tumor. They usually show central areas of necrosis surrounded by reactive gliosis.

Clinical Features

Symptoms depend on the site involved. They may cause headaches, dizziness, blurred vision, nausea and other symptoms.

Treatment

Radiotherapy is the primary treatment for brain metastases.

CHAPTER 12

Skeletal System

The skeleton is made-up of bones and cartilage. There are 206 bones in the human body. They are either flat, long, or tubular.

NORMAL STRUCTURE

Bone has two components:

1. *Cortical bone (compact bone)*: It is the dense outer shell consisting of haversian canals with blood vessels surrounded by concentric layers of mineralized collagen.
2. *Trabecular bone (cancellous bone)*: It is the bony trabeculae traversing the bone marrow (Fig. 12.1).

NORMAL HISTOLOGY

Bone has three types of cells namely, osteoblasts, osteocytes and osteoclasts.

1. *Osteoblasts*: They are the bone forming cells.
2. *Osteoclasts*: They are the bone resorbing cells.

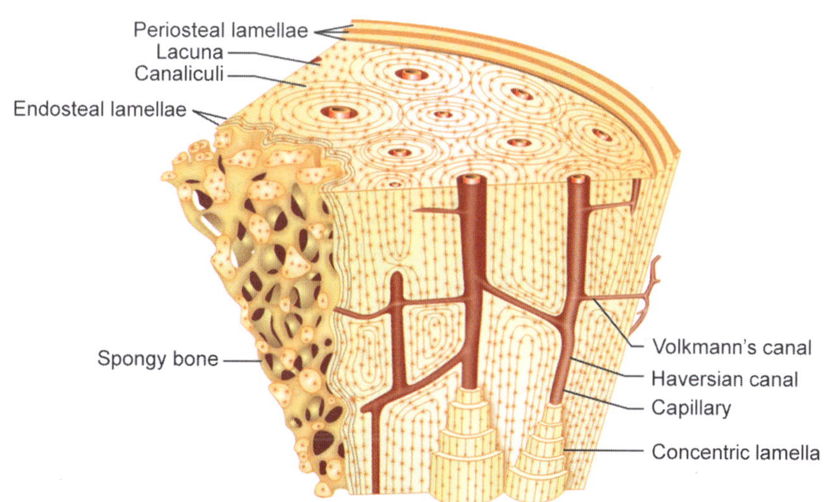

FIGURE 12.1 Diagrammatic representation of bone

3. *Osteocytes*: They are osteoblasts incorporated in the bone matrix.

Osteoid matrix: It consists of collagen type I and can be lamellar or woven.

Lamellar bone has parallel sheets of collagen fibers and has lesser number of small osteocytes. Woven bone has irregular and haphazard pattern of collagen fibers in bone matrix. It contains large number of closely packed osteocytes.

OSTEOMYELITIS

Osteomyelitis is the inflammation of the bone and marrow.

It can be divided into primary and secondary osteomyelitis. In primary osteomyelitis, there is a solitary focus of disease in the bone, whereas secondary osteomyelitis is the complication of any systemic infection.

Etiology

All types of organisms like bacteria, viruses, fungi and parasites can cause osteomyelitis. But pyogenic bacteria and mycobacteria are most common.

Pyogenic Osteomyelitis

It is caused by bacterial infection. *Staphylococcus aureus* is responsible in 90 percent of the cases. The other organisms involved are *E. coli, Pseudomonas, Klebsiella* and anaerobes. The most common route through which the infection spreads to bone is hematogenous route. It can also occur by direct implantation and extension from a contiguous site.

The location of the lesions in the bones varies with age. In the neonate, the infection of the metaphysis, epiphysis, or both can occur. In children, the metaphysis is affected. In adults, epiphysis and subchondral regions are also affected.

Pathologic Changes

The morphological changes depend on the duration, in respect to which it is classified into acute, subacute and chronic. Metaphysis is the most vascularized region of the bone. Bacteria gain access to the metaphysis through the nutrient arteries.

- Once the bacterium is localized in the bone, it proliferates and induces an acute inflammatory reaction. There is infiltration of neutrophils forming pus followed by cell death.
- The entrapped bone undergoes necrosis, following which the bacteria and inflammation spread along the marrow cavity, into endosteum, and then into haversian systems to reach the periosteum.
- The infection reaches the subperiosteal space forming subperiosteal abscess. It may penetrate through the cortex creating draining skin sinus tracts.
- Lifting of the periosteum further impairs the blood supply to the affected region which leads to bone necrosis. The dead piece of bone is known as the *sequestrum.*
- Subsequently, there is reactive bone formation at the site of inflammation and the new bone is called *involucrum.*

Clinical Features

It manifests as malaise, fever, chills, painful tender limb and leukocytosis. X-ray shows bony destruction.

Complications

- Septic arthritis
- Septicemia, endocarditis
- Pathological fractures
- Squamous cell carcinoma at the site of draining sinus tracts in long standing cases.
- Secondary amyloidosis in long standing cases
- Rarely sarcoma.

TUBERCULOUS OSTEOMYELITIS

Tuberculous osteomyelitis caused due to *M. tuberculosis* affects adolescents and young adults more often. It frequently involves spine (Pott's disease) and bones of extremities.

Pathological Changes

The bony lesion shows central caseous necrosis surrounded by tuberculous granuloma.

Pott's disease may be associated with compression fractures and destruction of intervertebral disks leading to paraplegia. Caseous material and pus extension from the lumbar vertebrae to the sheaths of psoas muscle leads to psoas abscess or lumbar cold abscess.

OSTEOPOROSIS

Osteoporosis is a disease associated with decreased bone mass. It is characterized by increased porosity of the skeleton. They are divided into primary and secondary osteoporosis:

Primary

- Senile osteoporosis
- Postmenopausal osteoporosis
- Idiopathic.

Secondary

Due to variety of causes like:

- Endocrine disorders like hyper and hypothyroidism, hyperparathyroidism, hypogonadism, type 1 diabetes, etc.
- Gastrointestinal disorders like malnutrition and malabsorption.
- Rheumatologic disease.
- Drugs like chemotherapeutic drugs, corticosteroids and anticonvulsants.
- Neoplasms like multiple myeloma.
- Miscellaneous causes being anemia, immobilization, osteogenesis imperfecta.

Pathogenesis

During young adulthood, there is peak bone formation. After the third or fourth decade, there is a slow bone resorption at a rate of 0.7 percent per year. Both males and females are equally affected. This is due to reduced physical activity, reduced synthetic activity of osteoblasts and reduced replicative activity of osteoprogenitor cells.

After menopause, there is decreased levels of estrogen and increased osteoclast activity which causes significant bone loss.

Pathology

In primary osteoporosis, the entire skeleton is involved. But vertebral bodies are more severely involved in postmenopausal osteoporosis. Microfractures are caused, which leads to vertebral collapse. Osteoporotic bones are brittle and are prone for pathological fractures. In old age, fracture of the head of the femur is common.

Clinical Features

Vertebral fractures are painful and multi-level fractures that cause height-loss and deformities like kyphoscoliosis and lumbar lordosis. Fracture of the femur neck and pelvis can cause complications like pulmonary embolism.

Prevention and Treatment

They include exercise, calcium and vitamin D intake and estrogen replacing agents in postmenopausal osteoporosis. Bisphosphonates and recombinant parathormone (PTH) are also in use.

FRACTURE HEALING

Fracture is defined as a disruption in the continuity of the bone. Healing of fracture depends upon the type of fracture. Fracture can be traumatic, where the underlying bone was previously normal or it may be a pathological fracture, where the bone was previously diseased. It can be a closed fracture where it is not exposed to outside or open where the skin above is disrupted. In simple fractures, there is a single fracture line whereas in comminuted or compound fractures, there are multiple bone fragments.

Fracture healing resembles skin wound healing to some extent. Two types of fracture unions are primary union and secondary union.

Primary union occurs when the fractured ends are approximated. Here there is formation of medullary callus. Periosteal callus formation is absent. Secondary union is very common. Here initially a procallus is formed followed by osseous callus and finally remodeling of the bone ends occur.

Procallus Formation

During procallus formation, the first step is formation of hematoma due to bleeding from the damaged blood vessels. A local inflammatory process begins at the fracture site followed by granulation tissue formation. The cells of the inner-layer of periosteum have osteogenic potential. They lay down collagen and osteoid matrix in this granulation tissue. This osteoid undergoes calcification and is then called woven bone callus. At times, cartilage can also be formed at the fracture site. Together the woven bone callus and the cartilage immobilize the fracture ends. Procallus is divided into external callus, which bridges the surface of the bone and internal callus, which bridges the medullary cavity.

Osseous Callus Formation

Osseous callus is composed of lamellar bone. The woven bone is resorbed by osteoclasts. New blood vessels develop and osteoblasts form osteoid.

Remodeling

Both osteoblastic and osteoclastic activity results in remodeling of the bone. External callus is removed and a bone marrow cavity develops in the internal callus. A compact bone indistinguishable from the normal bone is formed (Fig. 12.2).

Complications of Fracture Healing

- Nonunion occurs if soft tissue interposes between fracture ends.
- Delayed union occurs when there is old age, infection, foreign body, inadequate blood supply, denervation and improper immobilization.
- Fibrous union may occur if there is improper immobilization. A pseudo-joint may develop between the fracture ends.

BONE TUMORS

Bone tumors are broadly classified into primary and secondary bone tumors. Primary are those which arise from bones and secondary are metastases to bone from elsewhere. Primary bone tumors are further classified depending on the cell or tissue of their origin (Table 12.1).

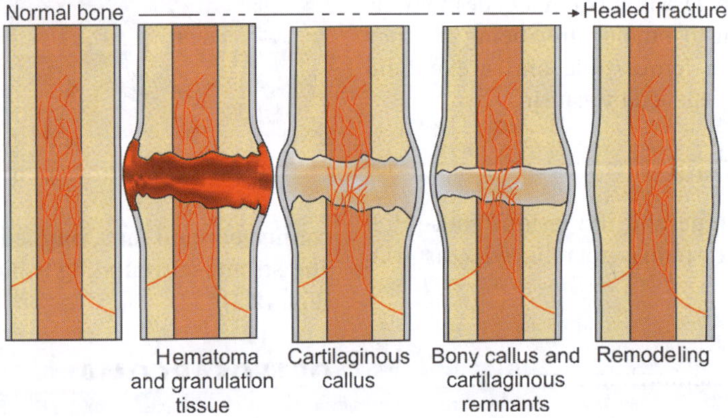

FIGURE 12.2 Diagrammatic representation of fracture healing

TABLE 12.1 Classification of primary bone tumors

Histologic type	*Benign*	*Malignant*
Osteogenic	Osteoid osteoma Osteoblastoma	Osteosarcoma
Chondrogenic	Osteochondroma Enchondroma Chondroblastoma Chondromyxoid fibroma	Chondrosarcoma
Hemopoietic	—	Myeloma Malignant lymphoma
Unknown origin	Giant cell tumor (Osteoclastoma)	Ewing's sarcoma Adamantinoma of long bones
Notochordal	—	Chordoma
Fibrogenic	Fibroma	Fibrosarcoma
Vascular	Hemangioma	Hemangioendothelioma Hemangiopericytoma
Lipogenic	Lipoma	Liposarcoma
Histiocytic	Fibrous histiocytoma	Malignant fibrous histiocytoma
Neurogenic	Neurilemmoma	Neurofibrosarcoma

OSTEOID OSTEOMA AND OSTEOBLASTOMA

They are closely related tumors and have similar histologic features. But they differ in their size, sites of origin and clinical symptoms.

Osteoid Osteoma

They are usually less than 2 cm, occur in young adults with male to female ration being 2:1. They are common in femur/tibia and are painful lesions. Pain is relieved by aspirin.

Osteoblastoma

They involve spine and the lesions cause dull achy pain and the pain is not relieved by aspirin.

Morphology

Gross: Both are hemorrhagic tan tissue.

Microscopy: They are composed of woven bone trabeculae which are haphazardly interconnected and are rimmed by osteoblasts. The stroma surrounding is highly vascularized (Fig. 12.3).

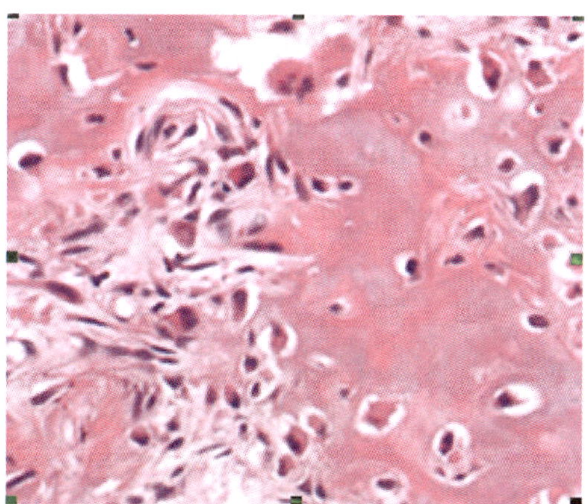

FIGURE 12.3 Microscopy of osteoblastoma

OSTEOSARCOMA

It is the most common primary malignant tumor of bone. It is a malignant mesenchymal

tumor in which cancerous cells produce bone matrix. It has bimodal age distribution. First peak occurs at ages younger than 20 years and the small second peak in the elderly. Men are more commonly affected than women. The tumors arise in the metaphyseal region of the long bones of the extremities.

Morphology

Gross

Tumors are gray white, gritty with areas of hemorrhage and cystic degeneration.

Microscopy

The tumor cells are pleomorphic and have hyperchromatic nuclei. Tumor giant cells and mitotic figures are commonly seen. Tumor cells produce neoplastic osteoid which have a coarse, lace like architecture (Fig. 12.4).

Clinical Features

They typically present as painful enlarging masses. X-ray shows lytic and blastic mass. The tumor lifts the periosteum. The triangular shadow in the X-ray between the cortex and raised ends of periosteum is known as Codman triangle.

They frequently metastasize to lungs, bones and brain. Treatment is surgery along with chemotherapy.

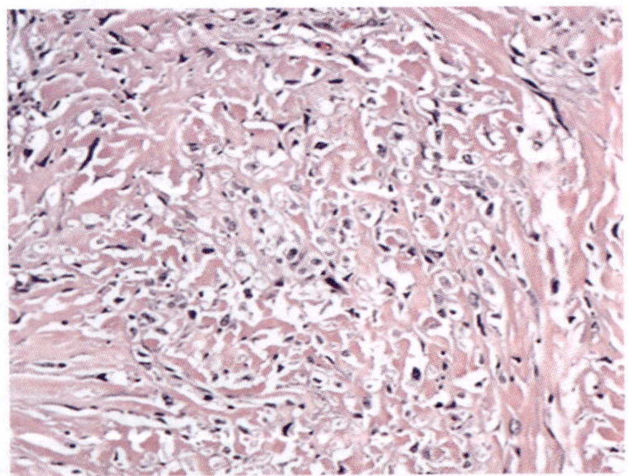

FIGURE 12.4 Microscopy osteosarcoma

CHONDROSARCOMA

These tumors produce neoplastic cartilage. They are common between 35 and 60 years of age. They are twice more common in men than women. Chondrosarcoma arise commonly in the central portions of the skeleton including pelvis, shoulder and ribs. They usually involve diaphysis of the bone.

Morphology

Gross

They are bulk tumors with grey white nodules. Cut surface show translucent, glistening tissue.

Microscopy

Depending on the level of differentiation of tumor cells, they are classified into grade 1, 2, 3 lesions. Low grade/grade 1 lesions show mild hypercellularity. Chondrocytes show vesicular nuclei and prominent nucleoli. Mitotic figures are rare. High grade/grade 3 tumors show increased hypercellularity, marked pleomor phism, tumor giant cells and increased mitotic figures (Fig.12.5).

Clinical Features

They present as painful enlarging masses. In X-ray, the more radiolucent the tumor, the greater the chances of it being high grade.

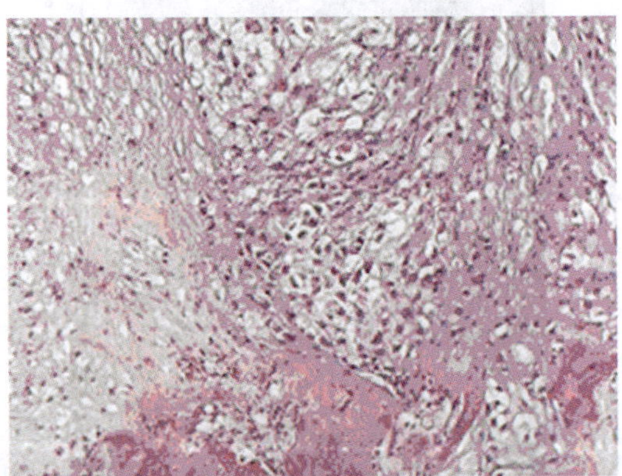

FIGURE 12.5 Microscopy of chondrosarcoma

Treatment is wide surgical excision with chemotherapy.

GIANT CELL TUMOR (OSTEOCLASTOMA)

It is a benign tumor but locally aggressive. It is common between 20 and 40 years of age and is believed to be from monocyte and macrophage lineage. Males and females are equally affected. They usually involve epiphysis and metaphysis. Majority of them arise around the knee (proximal tibia and distal femur).

Morphology

Gross

They are large, red brown tumors (Fig. 12.6).

Microscopy

Oval mononuclear cells are the proliferating component of the tumor. These have indistinct cell membranes. Increased mitosis is also seen. In the background, there are numerous osteoclast type of giant cells having multiple nuclei. The nuclei of these giant cells resemble those of mononuclear cells (Fig. 12.7).

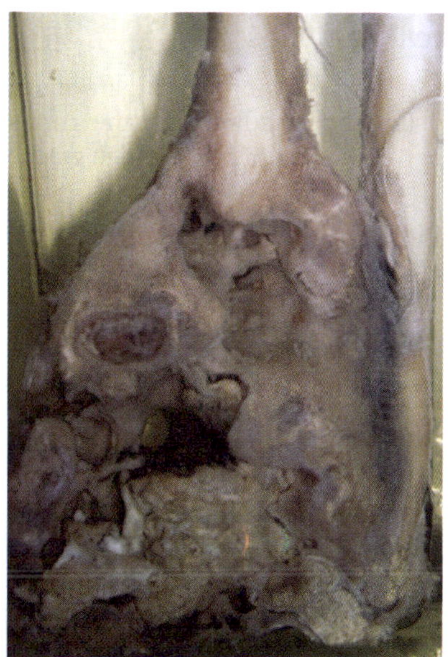

FIGURE 12.6 Gross photograph of osteoclastoma

Clinical Features

Since these tumors are close to joints, the patients may complain of arthritic symptoms. Rarely they present as pathological fractures. X-ray shows lytic, eccentric lesion with destruction of overlying cortex. Treatment is conservative surgery like curettage.

EWING'S SARCOMA

This tumor is a primary malignant small round cell tumor of bone. Similar tumor in soft tissue is called primitive neuroectodermal tumor (PNET). It is common between 10 and 15 years of age. Boys are more affected than girls. Ewing's sarcoma usually arises in the diaphysis of long tubular bones.

Morphology

Gross

They arise in the medullary cavity, invade the cortex and periosteum and produce a soft tissue mass. Tumor is tan-white with areas of hemorrhage and necrosis.

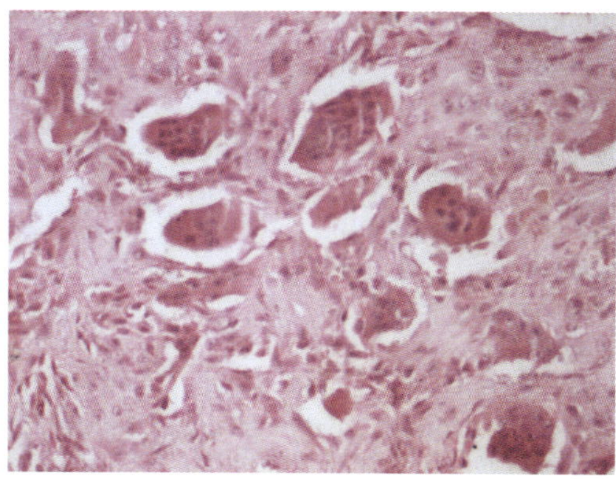

FIGURE 12.7 Microscopy of osteoclastoma

Microscopy

Sheets of uniform small round cells. These cells have scant cytoplasm. Some tumor cells are arranged in a circle about a central fibrillary space and are called *Homer-Wright rosettes* (Fig. 12.8).

Clinical Features

They present as painful, enlarging masses. The affected site is swollen and tender. Some patients have fever, anemia, increased WBC count and increased ESR all of which mimic infection. X-ray shows layers of reactive bone which appears as onion skin. Treatment is chemotherapy and surgical excision with or without radiation.

JOINTS

Joints are of two types. They are:

1. Solid or nonsynovial or synarthrodial joints.
2. Cavitated or synovial or diarthrodial joints.

Synovial joints have a joint space. There is a wide range of movements in these joints. The joint space is lined by synovial membrane which forms the synovial fluid that lubricates the joint during movements. Most of the diseases of the joints affect synovial joints.

Osteoarthritis

It is the most common type of joint disease and is characterized by progressive degenerative changes or progressive erosion of the articular cartilage.

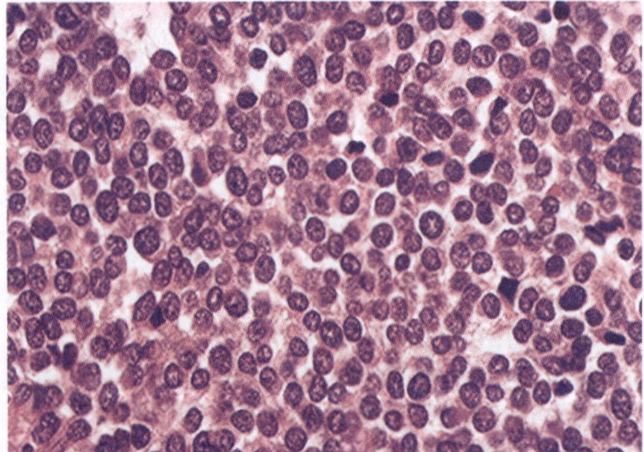

FIGURE 12.8 Microscopy of Ewing's sarcoma

They are of two types:

1. Primary
2. Secondary.

Primary Osteoarthritis

This is an aging phenomenon and is seen in the elderly. It is more common in the women than in men. Weight bearing joints, such as knee, hips and vertebrae are affected commonly.

Secondary Osteoarthritis

This can occur at any age and is due to wear and tear phenomena, repeated trauma to the joints, congenital deformities of the joint and other diseases like diabetes, obesity, etc. For example, knee joints are commonly affected in basketball players. In women, knee and hands are commonly involved, whereas hip involvement is common in men.

Morphology

Initially there is loss of cartilaginous matrix and chondrocytes. This is followed by vertical and horizontal fibrillation and cracking of the matrix. The articular surface becomes granular. Subsequently, the entire articular cartilage gets sloughed and subchondral bone below gets exposed. The exposed bone becomes smooth due to continuous friction and appears as polished ivory. Small fractures occur in this bone and pieces of it in the joint are then called joint mice. Synovial fluid enters into subchondral regions through these fracture gaps, gets loculated and form cysts. Bony outgrowths develop at the margins of articular cartilage and are called osteophytes. Synovium in advanced cases show chronic synovitis and hypertrophy of the villi.

Clinical Features

Minor osteoarthritis may be asymptomatic. Symptomatic cases present with deep, achy pain, which worsens with use, decreased mobility, stiffness of joints in the morning.

Osteophytes at the distal interphalangeal joints are characteristically seen in women and are called Heberden nodes.

In the spine, osteophytes can cause compression of cervical and lumbar nerve roots and cause radicular pain, muscular spasms and neurologic deficits.

Rheumatoid Arthritis

Rheumatoid arthritis is a chronic multisystem inflammatory disorder. It principally attacks the joints causing inflammatory arthritis. The other tissues and organs affected are blood vessels, heart, lungs, muscles and skin. It is common between 40 and 70 years of age and has a female preponderance.

Pathogenesis

The exact etiology is not known. It is believed to have an autoimmune etiology where a genetically susceptible host is exposed to an unknown antigen that is arthritogenic (Fig. 12.9).

Morphology

Small joints of the hands and feet, joints of wrists, elbows, ankles and knees are affected. Most commonly, involved joints are proximal interphalangeal and metacarpophalangeal joints.

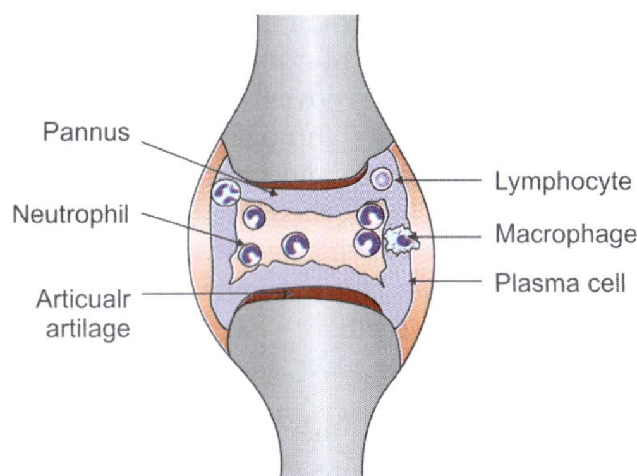

FIGURE 12.9 Diagrammatic representation of pathogenesis of rheumatoid arthritis

Grossly Synovium is Thickened and Edematous

Microscopy shows synovial stroma densely infiltrated by inflammatory cells like lymphocytes, plasma cells and macrophages along with increased vascularity and fibrinoid necrosis. There is formation of pannus which is a mass of synovium and synovial stroma consisting of inflammatory cells, granulation tissue and fibroblasts. This erodes the articular cartilage. Once the articular cartilage is destroyed, the pannus bridges the bones causing fibrous ankylosis, which finally results in bony ankylosis.

Extra-articular Lesions

Rheumatoid nodules are formed in the skin. They can also be seen in the spleen, lungs, pericardium, myocardium, aorta, heart valves and other organs. Blood vessels show acute vasculitis.

Clinical Features

The affected joints are swollen, painful and stiff in the morning. Destruction of joints causes deformities like radial deviation or wrist and ulnar deviation of fingers (swan neck deformity). X-ray shows loss of articular cartilage and joint space narrowing. Treatment consists of anti-inflammatory drugs and steroids.

Infectious Arthritis

Joints can become infected by all micro-organisms which reach them through blood.

Suppurative Arthritis

The common organisms involved are *Staphylococcus, Streptococcus, H. influenza, E. coli, Salmonella* and others. Predisposing factors are immunosuppression, IV drug abuse, trauma and chronic arthritis of other causes. Men and women are equally affected.

Pathology

The large joints like hip, knee, and ankle are commonly affected. Synovium becomes swollen and is infiltrated by neutrophils and mononuclear cells. An effusion develops in the joint space. Finally, fibrous adhesions are formed between the articular surfaces, which may result in bony ankylosis.

Tuberculous Arthritis

It is usually due to hematogenous dissemination from pulmonary infection or may develop as a direct spread from TB osteomyelitis. It is found commonly in children. The hip, knees and spine are commonly affected.

Pathology

It is usually monoarticular. The synovium shows granulomas with central caseous necrosis. Chronic disease causes fibrous ankylosis with joint space obliteration.

Gouty Arthritis

Gout is a disease characterized by hyperuricemia, which occurs due to disordered purine metabolism. The serum uric acid level is more than 7 mg/dL. Transient attacks of acute arthritis are seen due to crystallization of urates with in and about the joints.

Pathology

Acute synovitis occurs caused by precipitation of needle shaped crystals of monosodium urate from serum/synovial fluid. There is polymorphonuclear cell infiltration along with macrophages, which try to phagocytose these crystals. This aggregation of urate crystals surrounded by inflammatory cells like lymphocytes and macrophages is called tophi. Joint effusion is commonly seen. Chronic tophaceous arthritis causes fibrotic synovium resulting in fibrous or bony ankylosis.

Clinical Features

Asymptomatic hyperuricemia appears in males in puberty and after menopause in females. In acute arthritis that appears after several years, there is severe pain in the involved joint along with fever. It is seen affecting most commonly the great toe. Other joints affected are ankles, heels, knees, elbow, wrist and fingers.

CHAPTER 13

Hematology

Hematology is the study of blood. Blood constitutes a liquid portion called *Plasma,* in which formed elements, such as RBCs, WBCs and Platelets are suspended.

COLLECTION OF BLOOD

Blood can be collected by a skin prick method or venipuncture. For venipuncture, vacutainers are used nowadays.

Anticoagulants: Since many of the tests require blood which is not clotted, several anticoagulants are available to prevent clotting of blood. They are:

- Calcium chelaters:
  - Oxalate—potassium oxalate ammonium oxalate, balanced oxalate
  - Ethylene diamine tetra-acetic acid (EDTA)
  - Trisodium citrate.
- Heparin.

METHODS OF COLLECTION OF BLOOD FOR VARIOUS TESTS

Hematology

- Hemoglobin, TC, DC, platelets, peripheral smear-EDTA sample (1.5 mg/mL of blood).
- ESR by Westergren's method—trisodium citrate (3.8% solution)-anticoagulant. Ratio of citrate to blood = 1:4.
- Prothrombin time and activated partial thromboplastin time—citrate sample. Ratio of citrate to blood = 1:9.
- Osmotic fragility—heparinized blood.
- LE cell test—clotted blood.
- Sickling test—EDTA blood.
- Hb electrophoresis—EDTA blood.

Microbiology

For almost all routinely done tests like widal, VDRL, CRP, ASO titre, RA factor, TPHA, ANA, DsDNA, p-ANCA, c-ANCA, Hbs Ag, leptospira and dengue-clotted blood is used.

Biochemistry

- FBS, PPBS: Fluoride sample.
- Blood urea, serum creatinine, LFT: clotted blood.
- Hormones: T3, T4, TSH, progesterone, Prolactin, FSH, LH-clotted blood.
- Protein electrophoresis: clotted blood.

Hemoglobin Estimation

Hemoglobin is a molecule composed of four subunits, each containing a heme that is nestled in a hydrophobic crevice of a protein chain globin. The function of the hemoglobin is to carry oxygen from the lungs to the tissues, and to carry carbon dioxide back from the tissues to the lungs.

Hemoglobin concentration can be estimated by many methods under four principles:

1. Color measurement.
2. Iron content.
3. Specific gravity.
4. Oxygen combining capacity of blood.

Normal range of hemoglobin concentration in:

- Men: 13-16 g/dL
- Women: 11.5-15 g/dL.

METHODS OF ESTIMATION OF HEMOGLOBIN

- Colorimetric methods (measurement of color of hemoglobin or its derivative):
  - Talquist method
  - Sahli's method
  - Other methods—alkaline hematin method, Haldane method, Dare and Spencer methods.
  - Photometric methods—oxyhemoglobin or cyanmethemoglobin method.
- Physical method—specific gravity method.
- Chemical method—iron content measurement.
- Gasometric method—oxygen combining capacity measurement.

SAHLI'S METHOD OF ESTIMATION OF HEMOGLOBIN

Principle

In this method, hemoglobin is converted to acid hematin by the addition of N/10(0.1N) hydrochloric acid and the resulting brown color is compared with standard brown glass reference blocks. The intensity of brown color depends on the amount of acid hematin.

Sahli's Hemoglobinometer

It consists of standard brown glass blocks with a graduated tube. A special pipette called Sahli's pipette to measure 20 μL of blood is provided with this instrument. The graduated tube has markings in g percent (g/dL) on one side and percent of normal on the other (Fig. 13.1).

Method

N/10 HCl is prepared first by mixing 1 mL of concentrated HCl and 99 mL of distilled water. N/10 HCl is then taken into the graduated tube up to lowest mark. Blood is drawn up to 20 μL mark in Sahli's pipette and transferred into the tube. The acid and the blood is mixed by shaking the tube well and allowed to sit for at least 10 minutes for the brown color to develop. Then the solution is diluted with few drops of distilled water at a time, mixing well with the rod provided and then comparing the color of the fluid with the color of the comparator glass blocks, until the color matches. The rod is lifted up out of the solution when the color is being compared. The level of the fluid is noted at its lower meniscus and the corresponding reading on the scale in g/dL is given as the report.

Disadvantages

- Technical errors due to improper mixing.
- Methemoglobin, sulthemoglobin and carboxyhemoglobin are not converted to acid hematin.

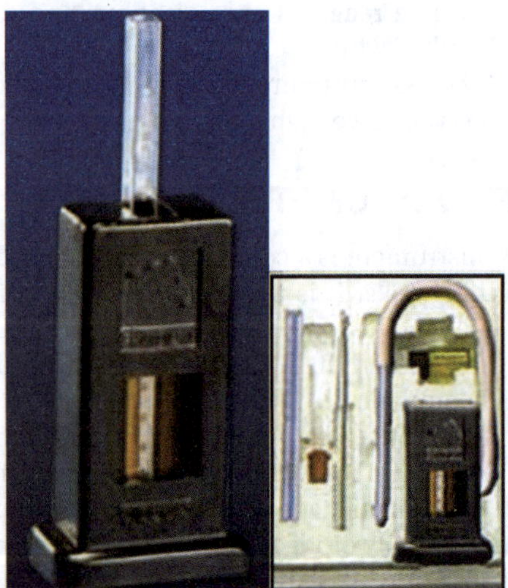

FIGURE 13.1 Sahli's hemoglobinometer

Cyanmethemoglobin Method

This method is used in many labs as it is most accurate.

Principle: The hemoglobin is first converted to methemoglobin by potassium ferricyanide and then to cyanmethemoglobin by sodium and potassium cyanide. The optical density of the solution is read in a spectrophotometer at 540 nm or using a yellow green filter.

The reagent used is: Drabkin's solution composed of:

- Dihydrogen potassium phosphate (anhydrous)
- Potassium ferricyanide
- Potassium cyanide
- Distilled water.

Method

About 5 mL of Drabkin's solution is taken into a cuvette. 20 μL of whole blood is added to it, mixed well and kept for 3 minutes. Then its absorbance readings are noted with the equivalent Hb value from the calibration curve or chart. The readings should always be taken against a reagent blank.

Disadvantages

- Cyanide reagents are poisonous and to be handled with care.
- Increased turbidity of blood like in leukocytosis can give higher absorbance readings.

HEMOCYTOMETER

This instrument is a counting chamber used for counting cells. It is accompanied by a pair of special pipettes, one called RBC pipette used for RBC count and the other WBC pipette used for WBC count.

The counting chamber with Neubauer ruling has two ruled stages separated by a small gutter. The two stages are separated by similar gutters from two ridges on either side, the upper surfaces of which are precisely 0.1 mm higher than the stages.

The large ruled area is 3 mm × 3 mm and includes nine square millimeters on each stage. Each large square is 1 mm square. The corner squares are each subdivided into 16 medium squares and are used for counting WBC. The center square is divided into 25 medium-size squares, each of which is in turn divided further into 16 small squares. The center square is used to count RBC (Figs 13.2A and B).

RBC Pipette

It has a bulb in which there is a small red glass bead. The lower part of the pipette is graduated with 10 marks below the bulb. The fifth-one from the tip is marked 0.5 and tenth-one is marked 1.0. There is one more line above the bulb, which is marked 101.

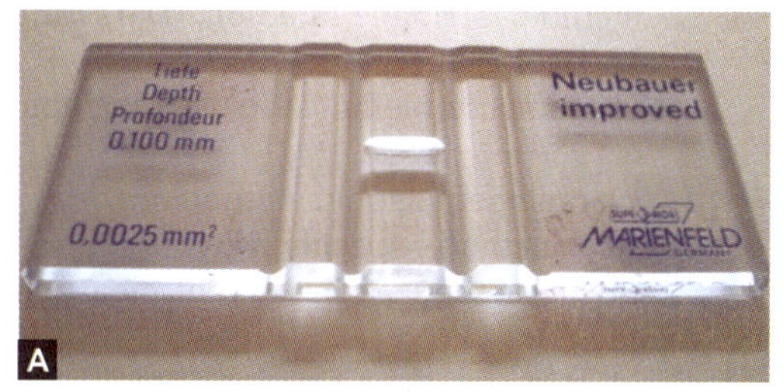

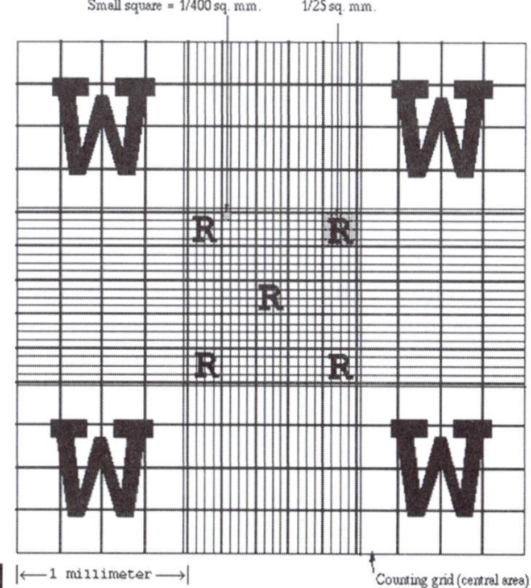

FIGURES 13.2A AND B (A) Neubauer chamber; (B) Neubauer ruling

WBC Pipette

The bulb in this has a white glass bead. The stem of the pipette has 10 marks, with 0.5 marked at the fifth line and 1.0 marked at tenth line. The line above the bulb is marked 11.

The beads in both the pipettes help in identification, mixing of the blood and the diluting fluid and help to know whether the pipette is dry enough.

THE RED BLOOD CELL COUNT

Method

Anticoagulated blood is drawn into RBC pipette upto 0.5 marks and then diluting fluid is drawn up until 101 marks above the bulb. This allows a dilution of 1: 200. The contents of the pipette are then well-mixed by rotating the pipette between the fingers horizontal to the axis of the pipette. The first few drops from the micropipette are discarded and then the tip of the pipette is placed on the platform of Neubauer chamber adjacent to the edge of the cover slip which is placed on the stage. The pipette is slightly inclined and pressure is released gently. A small volume of fluid is attracted and spreads under the cover slip by capillary action. There should be no air bubbles under the cover slip. The cells are allowed to settle down for 2 to 3 minutes and then they are counted under the microscope in all the squares of the entire central square.

RBC Diluting Fluid

There are many fluids like formal citrate solution, Dacie's formal citrate, normal saline, Hayem's fluid, Toisson's fluid and Gower's solution.

Calculation

$$\text{Number of cells}/\mu\text{L} = \frac{\text{Number of cells counted}}{\text{Dilution} \times \text{chamber depth} \times \text{chamber area}}$$

This is commonly expressed in

$$= \frac{\text{Cells} \times \text{dilution factor} \times \text{depth factor}}{\text{Area counted}}$$

$$\text{RBCs}/\mu\text{L} = \frac{\text{N} \times 200 \times 10}{1/5} = \text{N} \times 2000 \times 5$$

$$\text{RBCs}/\mu\text{L} = \text{N} \times 10000$$

The normal range of RBC count:

- *Male:* 4.5 million–6.5 million/cumm
- *Female:* 3.5 million–5.5 million/cumm

Increased RBC count is seen at birth, in hemoconcentration as in dehydration, severe burns, severe diarrhea or cholera, central cyanotic states, polycythemia vera.

Decreased RBC count is in anemia, childhood, old age and pregnancy.

TOTAL WHITE BLOOD CELL COUNT

Method of Estimation

Anticoagulated blood is drawn up to 0.5 marks of the WBC pipette and the diluting fluid is drawn up to 11 marks. This allows a dilution of 1:20. The pipette is well-shaken horizontally to its axis to mix the contents, and after discarding the first few drops, the counting chamber is charged as described for RBC count. The cells are counted under microscope in all the large corner four squares.

Diluting Fluid

The most commonly used diluting fluid is called Turke's fluid. It is composed of—glacial acetic acid, gentian violet stain and distilled water.

Calculation

$$\text{WBC}/\mu\text{L} = \frac{\text{Number of cells counted} \times \text{dilution factor} \times \text{depth factor}}{\text{Area counted}}$$

$$= \frac{\text{N} \times 20 \times 10}{4}$$

$$\text{WBCs}/\mu\text{L} = \text{N} \times 50$$

Normal range of total WBC count: 3500/µL–11000/µL.

Increase in the total count above 11000/µL is called leukocytosis and decreased total count below 3500/µL is called leukopenia.

Leukocytosis is seen in physiological causes such as:

- At birth, total count is high, often about 18000/μL
- Pregnancy
- Muscular exercise
- Heavy protein meal
- High fever, severe pain.

Pathological Causes

- Infections.
- Parasitic infestations.
- Severe trauma, hemorrhage and after surgery.
- Leukemia.

Causes of Leukopenia

- *Some infections like—Bacterial:* Typhoid, paratyphoid, tuberculosis. Viral: dengue, measles, etc. Protozoal: malaria.
- *Anemia:* Megaloblastic anemia.
- *Primary bone marrow depression:* Aplastic anemia.

DIFFERENTIAL WHITE BLOOD CELL COUNT

It is the number of different types of white cells present in the blood. They are counted by examining a well stained peripheral blood smear and expressed as percentage of total number of white cells counted. Usually 100 WBCs are counted.

Normal range of differential count :

- *Neutrophils:* 40–75%
- *Lymphocytes:* 30–45%
- *Monocytes:* 2–10%
- *Eosinophils:* 1–6%
- *Basophils:* 0–1%.

Platelet Count

To estimate platelet count, venous blood should always be used. Platelets normally disappear from blood at the site of injury by adhesion and aggregation, the reason why capillary blood (finger prick) is not the best specimen. The best anticoagulant that can be used is EDTA. It minimizes platelet adhesion and clumping.

Method of Estimation

About 20 μL of well-mixed EDTA blood is diluted with 1.98 mL of diluting fluid. This allows 1:100 dilution. It is well-mixed and the counting chamber is charged. The counting chamber is then kept in a petri dish with some moist paper to inhibit evaporation and is left for 10 minutes. The platelets will settle down in this time, so they will all be in the same plane of focus. Now the counting chamber is placed under the microscope and the platelets are counted in the central large square.

Calculation

$$\text{Platelets}/\mu\text{L} = \frac{\text{No. of cells counted} \times \text{dilution} \times \text{depth}}{\text{Area counted}}$$

$$= \frac{\text{N} \times 100 \times 10}{1}$$

$$\text{Platelets}/\mu\text{L} = \text{N} \times 1000$$

Normal range of platelet count: 1.5 to 4.5 lakhs/cumm.

Increase in the number of platelets above 4.5 lakhs/cumm is called thrombocytosis. It is seen in certain infections, immediately after hemorrhage, trauma or surgery. Decreased platelet count below 1.5 lakhs/cumm is seen in conditions like acute leukemia, aplastic anemia, megaloblastic anemia, hypersplenism, idiopathic thrombocytopenic purpura (ITP) etc.

BLOOD GROUPING AND TYPING

Grouping or typing a specimen of blood is the process in which a specific antisera is added to a suspension of the RBCs to find out which antigens are present in it. The blood groups are named for the antigens present on the RBCs.

ABO System

It is the most important of all the blood group systems.

Antigens and antibodies in ABO groups:

Group	Antigen on RBC	Antibody in serum
A	A	Anti-B
B	B	Anti-A
AB	A and B	None
O	Neither A nor B	Both Anti-A and Anti-B

Determination of Blood Group

Principle

This is based on slide agglutination. The RBCs have either A/B/both or none antigens. Suitable antibody is used for agglutination.

Procedure

A glass slide is cleaned with a gauze. It is marked 'A' at one side and 'B' at the other side. Antisera-A is placed on the side marked A and antisera-B is placed on the side marked B. RBC suspension to be tested is placed on both sides of the slide and are mixed with the respective antisera separately.

If the side marked A is agglutinated, then the blood group is 'A', similarly if side B is agglutinated, then it is 'B' group. If on both sides agglutination is seen, then 'AB' group and if not on both sides, it is 'O' group.

Rh (Rhesus) Typing

The most important Rh Ag is D antigen. Others are C and E.

Procedure to Determine Rh Group

A clean glass slide is taken and RBC suspension to be tested is placed on the slide. A drop of anti-D Rh antibody is added and mixed well. If there is agglutination, then it is Rh-positive. If there is no agglutination, then it is Rh-negative.

CROSS MATCHING

The procedure used to determine compatibility of donor and recipient blood is called the *cross match*. It is done in two parts, called the *major cross match* and *minor cross match*.

In the *major cross match*, the donor's cells are mixed with the patient's serum and in the *minor cross match*, the patient's cells are mixed with the donor's serum. A compatibility test is always very important to do before any transfusion.

Procedure: Coomb's Cross Matching

- Patient's and the donor's cells are washed three times in saline to remove all traces of serum. Then 5 to 10 percent suspensions of the cells are made in saline.
- Patient's tube is labeled (P) (major side). In this tube two drops of patient's serum and 2 to 3 drops of the donor cell suspension is taken.
- Donor's tube is labeled (D) (minor side). In this tube two drops of donor's serum and 2 to 3 drops of patient's cell suspension is taken.
- Both the tubes are incubated for one hour at 37°C.
- After one hour the tubes are centrifuged, serum is decanted and the cells are washed three times in saline.
- 1 to 2 drops of Coomb's serum is added to each tube, and after letting stand at room temperature for 5 minutes, the tubes are centrifuged slowly for 2 minutes.
- The cells are then examined both macroscopically and microscopically for agglutination.

The Coomb's serum in the cross match will detect the presence of immune antibodies, such as Rh antibodies and thus detect any Rh incompatibility. The major cross match is the most important. It does not require the lysis of many cells to produce a major transfusion reaction. The blood, which shows a major incompatibility should never be transfused.

The minor cross match is not as important as the major side. When minor incompatible blood is transfused, the donor plasma becomes diluted in the larger volume of the patient's plasma and so the donor antibodies become diluted and dispersed. There is no major reaction. But if many units are transfused within a short-period of time, then the antibodies will increase and reaction may occur.

TESTS FOR HEMOSTASIS

The process of stoppage of bleeding, forming a barrier to blood loss is called hemostasis. In Greek, "heme" means blood and "stasis" means to halt. The barrier mass is known as the blood clot, hemostatic plug or thrombus. Hemostasis involves a number of factors like platelets, plasma coagulation, fibrinolysis, anticoagulation protein systems and integrity of the vessel wall endothelium. Each of these balances the activities of the other.

Bleeding Time

It is the time taken for the bleeding to stop. Primary hemostasis is evaluated by the bleeding time. Factors affecting the bleeding time are platelet numbers, platelet function and vascular integrity.

Methods

- *Duke bleeding time:* Oldest methods where earlobe was punctured with a lancet.
- *Ivy bleeding time:* With BP cuff (40 mm Hg), incision is made on the forearm.
- *Template bleeding time:* Modification of ivy bleeding time.

In template bleeding time, a blood pressure cuff is placed on the patient's arm above the elbow and inflated to 40 mm Hg. A standardized horizontal incision is made on the volar surface of the forearm after cleaning the area with gauze using a glass or a plastic template which allows a blade to cut. A stopwatch is started and at 30 seconds intervals the blood is blotted away using filter paper. The bleeding time is the length of the time required for bleeding to stop.

Normal bleeding time: 1 to 9 minutes.

Prolonged bleeding time is seen in:

- When platelet count is low.
- Hereditary and acquired platelet dysfunctions.
- Von Willebrand disease.
- Afibrinogenemia and severe hypofibrinogenemia.
- When patient is using aspirin or aspirin like drugs.
- Some vascular bleeding disorders.

Clotting Time

It is the time taken for the freshly drawn blood to coagulate. It measures the integrity of intrinsic and extrinsic pathways of clotting. This test is rarely preferred nowadays as it is not very sensitive.

Methods

Modified Lee and White Method

There are many modifications of this test method. 3 to 5 mL of whole blood is drawn and about 1 to 1½ mL of blood is taken in three small test tubes, which are placed upright in a stand in a preheated waterbath maintained at 37°C for five minutes. Then gently the first of the tubes is tipped every 30 seconds to test for clotting and the time is recorded once it clots. The second tube is then tipped every 30 seconds and the time is recorded. The third tube is also treated the same way. The time recorded for clotting time of the third tube is taken as clotting time. (In this method, the purpose of the first two tubes is to tell us when to start looking at the third tube, the one in which there was least amount of disturbance.)

Some laboratories tip all the three tubes every 15 or 30 seconds and the average of the times taken for the three tubes to clot is reported as clotting time.

Capillary Tube Method

In this method, small sections of the blood filled capillary tubes are broken off at timed intervals and the time, when the blood strings

out between the broken surfaces is noted and taken as the clotting time.

Disadvantage: Capillary blood used is contaminated with tissue fluid from the injured tissue at the site of finger prick.

Normal clotting time: 8 to 15 minutes.

Prolonged clotting time is seen in:
- Clotting factors deficiency.
- Acquired bleeding disorders like disseminated intravascular coagulation (DIC).
- Circulating anticoagulants.

Prothrombin Time

It is the best screening test for abnormalities in the extrinsic pathway and common pathway of coagulation.

Method

The anticoagulant of choice is 3.8 percent sodium citrate. The ratio of anticoagulant to whole blood is 1:9. The citrated whole blood is centrifuged to separate plasma from cells.

To the plasma, an optimal concentration of tissue thromboplastin is added. After a brief incubation at 37°C, calcium chloride is added to the mixture and the time required for a clot to form is measured.

Normal prothrombin time: 11 to 15 seconds.

Prolonged prothrombin time is seen in:
- Factors I, II, V, VII, X deficiency.
- Obstructive jaundice.
- Vitamin K deficiency.
- During coumarin anticoagulant treatment.
- Heparin administration.
- In 75% of patients with DIC.
- In dysproteinemias.

EXAMINATION OF BONE MARROW

Hematopoiesis

In the few weeks of gestation, yolk sac is the main site of hematopoiesis in the human embryo. Liver and spleen are the main sites by third month of gestation and remains so until about 2 weeks after birth.

Hematopoiesis begins in the bone marrow by 4th or 5th month of gestation. During childhood, there is progressive fatty replacement in the marrow of long bones and the hematopoietic marrow in the adult life is confined to vertebrae, sternum, skull, ribs, pelvis and sacrum.

The developing cells in the bone marrow are present outside the marrow sinuses. On maturation, they enter the marrow sinuses, microcirculation and from there released into circulation.

Examination

It is of a great value in confirmation of clinical diagnosis or that suspected on peripheral blood film. A peripheral blood smear examination must, therefore, always be done before bone marrow examination.

Bone marrow can be examined by four techniques:
- Bone marrow aspiration
- Bone marrow biopsy (core biopsy)
- Open biopsy
- At autopsy.

Indications for bone marrow aspiration:
- Decreased blood cell counts like anemia, leukopenia, thrombocytopenia and pancytopenia.
- In leukemias (acute and chronic) and lymphomas.
- In storage disorders like Gaucher's disease.
- Infections
  - In case of disseminated tuberculosis.
  - In Kala-azar, a disease caused by *leishmania donovani.*
  - Other parasitic infestations and fungal infections.
- In multiple myeloma
- Unexplained enlargement of liver and spleen.
- Suspected tumor infiltration into marrow.
- PUO (pyrexia of unknown origin).
- To assess iron stores.

Indications for Bone Marrow Biopsy

- 'Dry tap' where there is failure to obtain marrow particles from aspiration. It usually occurs in conditions like:
  - Aplastic anemia
  - Myelofibrosis
  - Packed marrow/metastasis
  - Procedural failure
- Hairy cell leukemia
- Osteopetrosis.

Sites of Bone Marrow Sampling

- Posterior superior iliac spine
- Anterior superior iliac spine
- Tibia
- Sternum
- Vertebral spinous process/ribs (Fig. 13.3).

Bone Marrow Needles

- Salah needle—used for aspiration.
- Klima needle—used for aspiration.
- Jamshidi needle—used for both aspiration and biopsy (Fig. 13.4).

Procedure

Aspiration

Performed with all aseptic precautions. Overlying skin is cleaned. In adults, posterior superior iliac spine or sternum is the usual sites. In infants below 2 years of age, the front end of tibia is used. After injecting a small dose of local anesthetic drug to anesthetize the skin and the periosteum, the bone marrow needle, either Salah or Klima is taken and inserted into the bone marrow. The stilette is withdrawn and a 10 cc syringe is attached to aspirate around 0.2 to 0.5 mL of marrow. Immediately, it is taken onto clean glass slides and smears are made. These smears can be stained with Leishman stain or Wright's stain for interpretation (Fig. 13.5).

Advantage of Aspiration

Individual cell morphology is better assessed than in biopsy.

Trephine Biopsy

Performed by Jamshidi needle by which a core of tissue from periosteum to bone marrow cavity

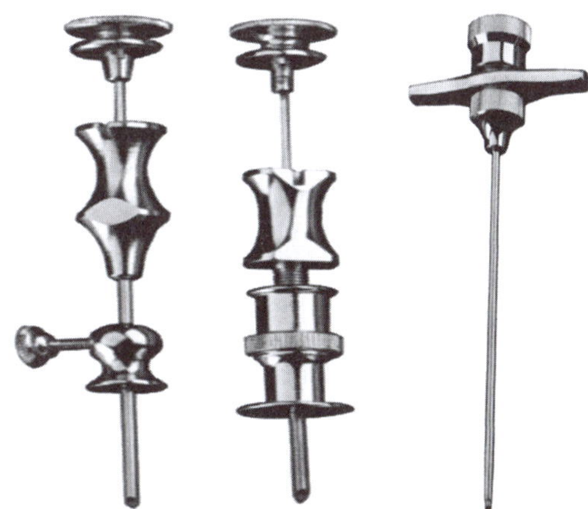

FIGURE 13.4 Salah, Klima and Jamshidi bone marrow needles

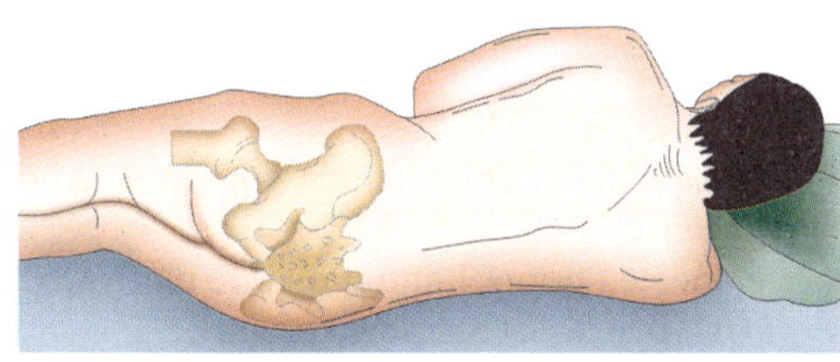

FIGURE 13.3 Bone marrow sampling site

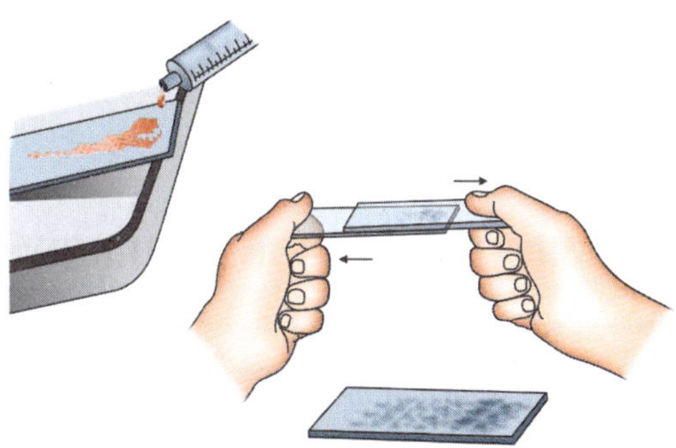

FIGURE 13.5 Smear making

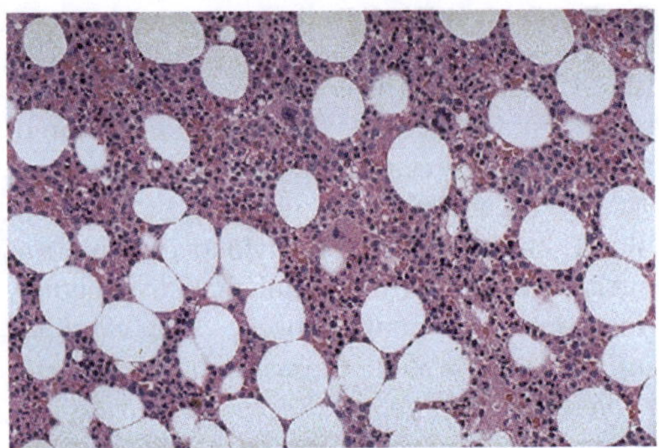

FIGURE 13.6 Microscopy of bone marrow biopsy showing cells and marrow fat

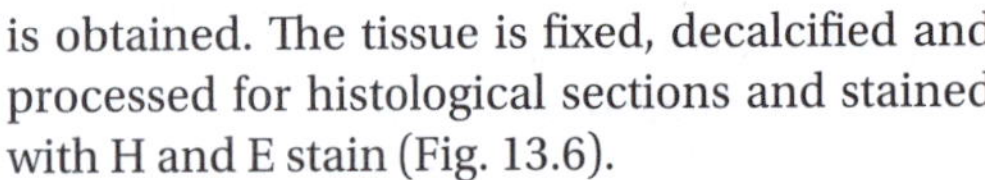

is obtained. The tissue is fixed, decalcified and processed for histological sections and stained with H and E stain (Fig. 13.6).

Advantage of Biopsy

Excellent view of overall architecture, cellularity and infiltration.

Interpretation

Bone marrow is evaluated under following headings:

- *Cellularity:* Normocellular or hypercellular or hypocellular.
- *Cell: fat ratio:* Ratio of hemopoietic elements to marrow fat.
- *Myeloid:* Erythroid ratio (M:E ratio)- Normal = 2 or 3 : 1.
- *Erythropoiesis:* Maturation—normoblastic or megaloblastic or micronormoblastic and evidence of dyserythropoiesis.
- *Myelopoiesis:* Maturation and evidence of dysmyelopoiesis.
- *Megakaryopoiesis:* Any alteration in numbers and evidence of dysmegakaryopoiesis.
- *Accessory cells:* Lymphocytes, plasma cells, osteoblasts and histiocytes (storage cells).
- Granulomas or parasites or any metastatic deposits (Fig. 13.7).

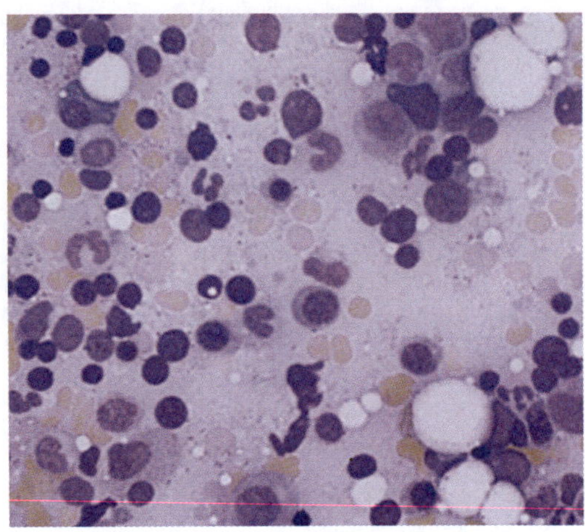

FIGURE 13.7 Bone marrow smear

Differential Count

A good focus of smear is selected and a 500 cell count is done.

- Myeloblast—(0-3)
- Promyelocyte—(3-12)
- Myelocyte (N)—(2-13)
- Metamyelocyte and band forms—(8-12)
- Neutrophils—(22-46)
- Myelocytes (eo)—(0-3)
- Eosinophils—(0.3-4)
- Basophils—(0-0.5)
- Monocytes—(0-3)
- Plasma cells—(0-3.5)
- Erythroblasts—(5-35)
- Megakaryocytes—(0-2)
- Lymphocytes—(5-20) and macrophages—(0-2).

Special Stains

- Perls's stain is done for aspiration smears to assess the iron stores in the marrow (Fig. 13.8).
- Reticulin stain is done for biopsy slides to quantify marrow reticulin (Fig. 13.9).

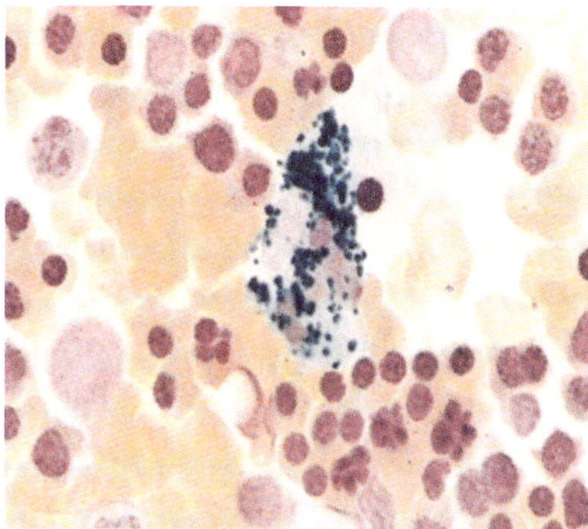

FIGURE 13.8 Perls' stain to assess iron stores

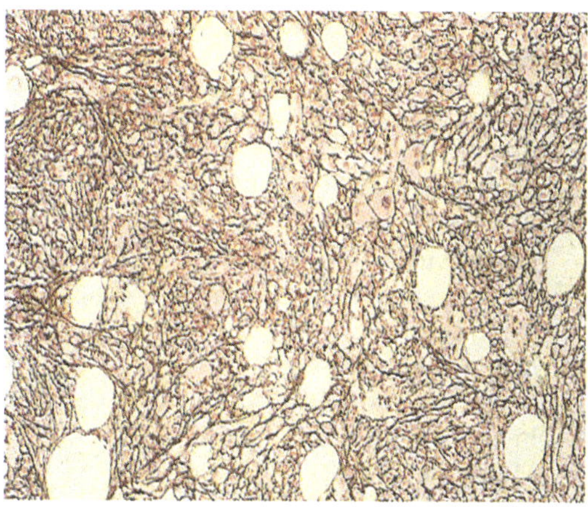

FIGURE 13.9 Reticulin stain of bone marrow biopsy to assess marrow reticulin

BLOOD CULTURE

Blood for culture is probably the most important specimen, which helps the prompt initiation of specific therapy against the offending organism.

The organisms most likely to be found in blood cultures are: staphylococci, coliform bacilli, α and α haemolytic streptococci, pneumococci, enterococci, *Haemophilus influenza, Brucella, Clostridium perfringens, Proteus, Pseudomonas, Bacteriodes, Neisseria, Salmonella, Leptospira,* etc.

The media used are:

- 50 mL of brain heart infusion broth
- Bile broth.

Anaerobic media such as:

- Thioglycollate broth
- Robertson's cooked meat medium.

Collection of Blood

The skin is cleaned with spirit and iodine. The needle and the top of the bottle are flamed before inoculating 5 mL of blood into each culture bottle. The mouth of each culture bottle is flamed again before the cover is replaced.

The cultures are immediately placed in the incubator overnight, in 5 percent CO_2 sub cultures are made every 2 days until growth is seen or until 2 weeks. Only after 2 weeks, if there is no growth, "No Growth" report can be sent. When bacterial endocarditis or brucellosis is suspected the report is given after 3 weeks.

CHAPTER 14

Examination of Body Cavity Fluids, Transudates and Exudates

CEREBROSPINAL FLUID ANALYSIS

Cerebrospinal fluid (CSF) is an ultrafiltrate of plasma which is found between the arachnoid and pia mater and surrounds the brain and spinal cord.

Methods of Specimen Collection

Lumbar Puncture

The lumbar puncture needle is a long thin needle with a stiletto snugly fitting into the 1-1.5 mm bore of the needle (Fig. 14.1).

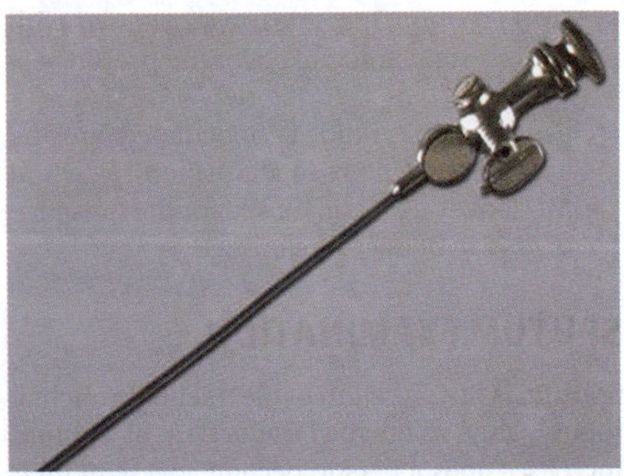

FIGURE 14.1 Photograph of a lumbar puncture needle

Site

The site for lumbar puncture is between the 3rd and the 4th lumbar vertebrae after administering the local anesthetic. Once the needle is inside the subarachnoid space, the stilette is withdrawn and the CSF is collected and sent for analysis.

Examination of CSF

The CSF must be examined, as early as possible, within 30 minutes of receiving the sample in the laboratory.

- *Color:* Usually, CSF is colorless. If it is red in color, it indicated that it is a traumatic tap. Yellowish discoloration of CSF called xanthochromia is seen in subarachnoid hemorrhage after some days.
- *Turbidity:* Normally CSF is clear. Cloudiness or turbidity is seen in case of pyogenic meningitis.
- *Cytology:* Normally, CSF contains very few cells 0–5 WBCs/μL. No RBC is seen usually. Due to the scanty cellularity, CSF is counted undiluted. The undiluted sample is charged in the Neubar's counting chamber and all the 9 squares are counted. The total number of cells counted is given as the cell count/μL.
- *Differential WBC count:* The CSF is centrifuged and the sediment is made into

smears, stained with Giemsa or Wrights stain and studied. The number of lymphocytes and neutrophils are counted and given as percentage.

- Biochemical examination of the amount of protein and sugar present is estimated by chemical tests.
- The level of chloride is estimated.
- *Microbiological examination:* The fluid is inoculated in the appropriate culture media of blood agar and McConkey agar and looked for the presence of growth of microorganisms.

CAVITY FLUID EXAMINATION

The most commonly examines cavity fluids are pleural fluid and peritoneal fluid (ascitic fluid).

Collection of Specimen

Pleural fluid is collected by puncturing the pleural cavity in the intercostals spaces under aseptic precautions.

Peritoneal fluid is obtained by ascitic/peritoneal tap where a needle is introduced into the peritoneal cavity aseptically.

Both the fluids should be transferred to the laboratory as early as possible for examination.

Table 14.1 lists the differences between transudate and exudate.

TABLE 14.1 Differences between Transudate and exudate

Character	*Transudate*	*Exudate*
Appearance	Clear	cloudy
Color	Straw-yellow	Yellow to red
Odor	None	May have, if septic
Specific gravity	Less than 1.018	More than 1.018
Protein	Less than 2.0 g/dL	More than 2.0 g/dL
Glucose	10–20 mg/dL	May be very low
Cells	Low count	High count
Bacteria	None	May be present

Protocol for the examination of cavity fluids:

- *Volume:* Record the volume of the fluid received in a measuring jar.
- *Appearance:* Note the color, appearance (clear/cloudy), odor of the fluid.
- *Protein and glucose:* These are measured by chemical tests.
- *Cell count:* The fluid is drawn till the 0.5 mark in the WBC diluting pipette. Then, the WBC diluting fluid is drawn till the mark 11. After proper mixing, the Neubar's counting chamber is charged. Counting is done in the 4 corner WBC squares, under the 40x objective.

$$\text{No. of cells}/\mu\text{L} = \frac{\text{Total no. of cells counted in 4 squares}}{\text{Chamber depth} \times \text{dilution} \times \text{area counted}}$$

$$= \frac{N \times 10 \times 10}{4}$$

No. of cells/μL = N × 50

- *Cell type:* The fluid is centrifuged and the smears are made of the sediment. The smears are stained with Leishman's or Wright's stain and examined under the microscope. The percentage of lymphocytes, neutrophils and mesothelial cells are noted.
- *Cytology for malignant cells:* The smears are stained with Papanicolaou stain and looked for the presence of malignant cells.
- *Gram's stain:* The smears are stained with Gram's stain and looked for the presence of bacteria.
- *Culture:* The fluid is inoculated in the appropriate culture media of blood agar and McConkey agar and looked for the presence of growth of microorganisms.

SPUTUM EXAMINATION

Sputum is the secretion of the tracheobronchial tubes. Only when the production of sputum increases does a person become aware of their presence. The excess of sputum is evacuated by coughing.

Collection of Sputum

Patients are instructed to collect only material coughed up from the trachea and not the saliva from the mouth. Usually an early morning specimen is sufficient. It is collected in closable cups or wide mouthed bottles with covers.

Macroscopic Examination

- *Quantity or volume:* The quantity of sputum coughed up in 24 hours is examined. It varies with different diseases. Cough can be dry (nonproductive) or productive.
- *Consistency:* It can be serous, frothy, mucoid, purulent, seropurulent or hemorrhagic.
- *Odor:* Sputum is usually odorless. It can be foul in conditions like lung abscess.
- *Color:* It may be colorless. The presence of pus gives it a whitish yellow color. In smokers, it becomes grayish black. When blood is present in the sputum, it is called 'hemoptysis'. The hemoglobin when gets altered with the passage of time, sputum becomes reddish brown. This is called 'rusty sputum'.
- *Other findings:* Bronchial casts, broncholiths (lung stones), sulfur granules, parasites and foreign bodies.

Microscopic Findings

- *Unstained sputum:* It is examined to look for:
  - *Elastic fibers:* Indicates destructive process in the lungs.
  - *Curschmann's spirals:* Wiry spiral structures seen in sputum of patients with bronchial asthma.
  - *Charcot-Leyden crystals:* Fine, needle shaped or hexagonal, colorless crystals seen in patients with bronchial asthma.
  - *Pigmented cells:* Macrophages showing dark brown blood pigment (hemosiderin) can be seen.
  - *Fungi:* Colonies of fungi may be seen.
  - *Parasites:* Parasitic worm larvae are rarely seen.
- *Stained sputum smear:* Sputum smears are made on dry, clean slides. They are fixed over a flame and stained with Gram's stain and Ziehl-Neelson stain for bacteria. Papanicolaou stain can also be done to look for the presence of tumor cells. Wright's stain or Leishman stain may be used to see various cells like neutrophils, eosinophils, lymphocytes, mononuclear cells, epithelial cells and RBCs (Fig. 14.2).

Sputum Culture

Culture is done to study various bacteria and fungi.

GASTRIC ANALYSIS

Gastric juice has to be examined to know about the functions of the stomach. Examination of a fasting specimen and then examination of gastric juice obtained after stimulation of gastric mucosa is done.

Obtaining Gastric Juice

Gastric juice is obtained by aspiration through a Ryle's tube which is inserted through the pharynx and esophagus down into the stomach. It is collected in the morning after the patient has fasted (has not taken any fluid or food by mouth) for the previous 12 hours.

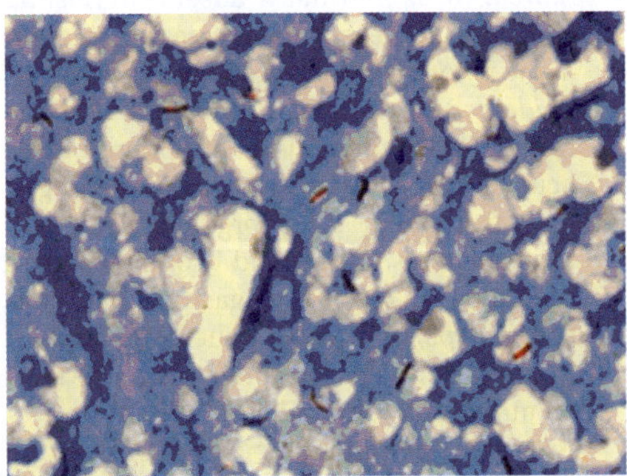

FIGURE 14.2 Ziehl-Neelsen staining of sputum showing acid fast bacilli

Stimulants of gastric secretion: More recently, the stimulation is done by an injection of histamine or one of the analogs of the hormone 'gastrin'. This does not require the addition of any substances into the stomach during the test. Collection of poststimulation specimens is done by continuous suction applied to the gastric tube.

Examination of Gastric Juice Specimens

- *Volume:* Normal fasting gastric juice is around 20 to 50 mL. It may go up to 100 mL. Volume in excess of 100 mL is abnormal.
- *Color:* Normally it is colorless. If there is any bile regurgitation, it becomes green in color. Bleeding makes it red, or brown when blood is older.
- *Consistency:* Normally it is watery. Food particles if present in the fasting specimen indicate obstruction to the outflow or decreased motility.
- *Odor:* It is odorless but fermentation or putrefaction makes it foul.
- *Reaction:* It is normally acidic. pH strips or pH meters can be used to measure it.
- *Mucus:* It can be seen as jelly like substance in the gastric juice. In conditions like gastritis it is seen in large quantities.
- *Blood:* Presence of blood is called 'hematemesis'.
- *Starch:* It is normally absent in fasting specimen. If present, it indicates obstruction at the pylorus or decreased motility.
- *Acidity:* Both free acid and total acid are tested. HCl is the major component of free acid. Total acid includes HCl, hydrogen ions from acid salts, organic acids and mucoproteins. If free acid is of a value less than 10 mL/100 mL of gastric juice, it is called *hypochlorhydria*. When the amount in any one of the specimens is more than 60 ml/100 mL, it is called *hyperchlorhydria* if is often seen in peptic ulcer. When none of the specimens show any free acid, it is called *achlorhydria.* When it is absent even after stimulation with histamine, it is called 'Histamine fast achlorhydria' which is most commonly seen in pernicious anemia.
- *Bacteria:* Gram's stain is done for a smear made out of centrifuged deposit of gastric juice. Normally there is no bacteria in gastric juice. It may be seen in gastric obstruction.
- *Cytology:* Papanicolaou staining is done to identify tumor cells which may have been exfoliated into the gastric juice.

SEMEN ANALYSIS

Indications of semen analysis:

- Investigation of infertility
- To check on the completeness of vasectomy
- In medicolegal cases to settle the cases of disputed paternity.

The production of seminal fluid is by the seminal vesicles, the prostate and the Cowper's glands. It serves as a medium to hold the spermatozoa.

Specimen Collection

The person has to abstain from sex for a period of 4 days. The sample is collected by masturbation into a clean, dry wide mouthed bottle. It should be transported to the laboratory as soon as possible, preferably within 30 minutes.

The freshly ejaculated semen is highly viscous. It must liquefy which usually occurs in 15 to 30 minutes and is due to the action of enzymes in the seminal fluid. Once the liquefaction occurs, the semen must be examined immediately.

Macroscopic Examination

Volume: Normal volume ranges from 2.5 to 5 mL.

Viscosity: Freshly ejaculated semen is highly viscous. Self-liquefaction should be completed within 30 minutes.

Color: Normal semen is opaque or cloudy.

Microscopic Examination

Motility: Place a drop of liquefied semen on a glass slide, cover the drop with a cover slip and rim the edges of the cover slip with Vaseline to prevent evaporation and drying. Examine fewer than 40x (high power) objective. Normally, many sperms will be moving in all directions. Note the percentage of actively motile, sluggishly motile and nonmotile sperms. Normally at least 80 percent of sperms will be actively motile. Decreased motility of less than 20 percent would suggest infertility.

Sperm count: After liquefaction, take the semen in the WBC pipette up to '0.5' mark and then draw in the semen diluting fluid up to the mark '11'. Mix well. This will give a dilution of 1:20 and a dilution factor of 20. The semen diluting fluid contains sodium bicarbonate, phenol and distilled water. The sodium bicarbonate counteracts the mucus and allows even dilution; phenol kills the sperms and stops the movement so that they can be counted.

Charge the Neubar's counting chamber (with a depth of 0.1 mm) and count the number of sperms in four corner WBC squares.

$$\text{Sperms/mL} = \frac{\text{No. of sperms counted} \times 1000}{\text{Dilution} \times \text{chamber depth} \times \text{chamber area}}$$

$$= \frac{N \times 20 \times 10 \times 1000}{4}$$

Sperms/mL = N × 50,000

The normal sperm count as 15–150 million/mL (According to the WHO criteria 2010).

Patients with a count less than 60 million/mL are said to have *oligospermia*. Patients with low count and reduced motility are said to have *oligozoospermia*. Patients with sperm count less than 15 million/mL are said to have oligozoospermia.

Condition with no sperms in the semen is called *azoospermia*. Patients with low sperm count and reduced motility are said to have oligoasthenospermia.

Morphology: To study the morphology, the liquefied semen is made into a smear and stained with Leishman stain or aqueous basic fuchsin. The abnormalities include double headed sperms, absence of neck, short tail, double tail or absent tail. In normal semen, the abnormal forms should not be more than 20 percent.

CHAPTER 15

Examination of Urine and Feces

INTRODUCTION

Urine is the ultrafiltrate of plasma. It is one of the most easily obtained specimens examined in laboratory. Urine examination gives us information about the functioning of the kidneys and possible abnormalities of urinary tract and may also lead to the diagnosis of various systemic diseases of human body which are reflected by the presence of various substances in urine.

FORMATION OF URINE

Urine is formed in the kidneys as the product of ultrafiltration of plasma by renal glomeruli, followed by reabsorption of most of the water and some of the solute in the tubules, as well as by active secretion of some substances by tubular epithelium. Then the urine is collected and passed on down from the kidneys through the ureters for temporary storage in the urinary bladder pending final passage to the outside of the body through urethra.

COLLECTION OF URINE

For routine examination any fresh specimen of urine is adequate. It is best collected as an early morning specimen is voided, when the patient first wakes up from a night's sleep as it is the most concentrated single specimen and it has the lowest pH. It tends to preserve the formed elements well.

A 24-hour specimen is needed for quantitative tests and for concentration of tubercle bacilli. It is collected by discarding the early morning urine specimen and then all the urine voided in the day up to next day morning is included.

Under normal conditions there is little variation in the urine composition from day to day in 24 hours specimens, but there may be great difference in single specimens taken at various times during the day depending on the amount of water intake, dietary intake, drinks like coffee or tea.

Specimens for bacteriological examination have to be collected with utmost care to prevent contamination in a sterile container. It is the mid-stream specimen [after first several mL have rinsed out the terminal urethra]. Then glans penis in the male or the anterior vulva in the female have been carefully cleansed , without touching the lip of the container to the skin surface, the urine sample is collected. This is called the clean catch specimen. Quantitative assessment of bacteriologic growth in the cultured urine can yield differentiation between significant and insignificant levels of growth.

Preservation of Urine

In general, early morning or random specimen should be examined within 1 to 2 hours after

the patient has voided. If there is delay, then the specimen should be refrigerated. When 24 hours specimens are being collected or when a sample has to be transported or mailed to a distant laboratory for examination, it is necessary to add preservatives to the urine to prevent decomposition and growth of the contaminating organisms. Commonly used preservatives are:

- Toluene—best all round preservative and is added in sufficient quantity to form a thin layer on the surface of the urine.
- Boric acid—in preparation of 5 g per 4 oz is added to about 120 mL of urine.
- Concentrated hydrochloric acid—10 mL per 24 hours specimen.
- Formalin and chloroform—one drop per 30 mL of urine is used.
- Thymol—one crystal to the specimen of urine is added.

Macroscopic Examination

Volume

Normal range of urine volume is 1.2–2 L/day.

Increased excretion of urine of more than two liters per day is called *polyuria*. It is seen physiologically in cold weather, after high intake of fluids and when on diuretic therapy. Pathologically it is seen in diabetes insipidus, diabetes mellitus, and Addison's disease.

Decreased excretion of urine of less than 500 mL/day is called *oliguria*. It is seen physiologically in hot weather and with reduced fluid intake. Pathologically oliguria is seen in chronic renal failure, prolonged diarrhea, vomiting, excess sweating, severe burns and in acute tubular necrosis.

Anuria refers to total absence of urine, seen in end stage renal disease.

Nocturia is excretion by an adult of urine more than 500 mL at night.

Color

Normally, urine is straw colored. This color is due to urochromes and small amount of urobilin that are present in urine. Change in the color of urine is seen in different conditions. Some of the examples are given below:

- *Reddish brown:* Due to increased urobilinogen or porphyrins.
- *Bright red:* Due to large amount of fresh blood in urine.
- *Pink:* Due to small amount of blood in urine.
- *Brown:* Due to blood pigments.
- *Brownish yellow or green:* Due to bile pigments.
- *Milky white:* Seen in chyluria due to filarial infestation.
- *Orange:* During treatment with rifampicin.

In porphyria, urine turns dark brown on exposure to sunlight.

Odor

Freshly passed urine has slight aromatic odor. If allowed to stand, it emits ammoniacal smell because of decomposition of urea and liberation of ammonia gas.

Presence of ketone bodies in urine produces fruity odor.

Appearances

Normally, urine is clear. It may become cloudy due to the presence of amorphous phosphates. Amorphous urates in acid urine disappear on heating.

In disease, urine may be cloudy due to the presence of:

- Many pus cells
- Bacteria or fungi
- Suspension of fat or chyle.

Reaction

Normally, the pH of urine ranges between 4.6 and 8.0, usually slightly acidic. A pH of 6.0 is due to the presence of various acid ions, such as sulfates, chlorides and some organic acids.

As urine stands at room temperature, it becomes alkaline.

The reaction is measured by using litmus paper. In acid urine, red litmus turns blue. In

alkaline urine, red litmus becomes blue. In neutral urine, both red and blue turn purple.

Acidic urine is seen in ketosis, systemic acidosis and acidification therapy.

Alkaline urine is seen in *Pseudomonas* infection, systemic alkalosis and on alkali therapy.

Specific Gravity

Specific gravity of urine gives an indication of the amount of solids in the solution.

Normal specific gravity of urine is 1.015 to 1.025 in a 24-hour urine sample.

Chief substances that influence the specific gravity of urine are urea, sodium, calcium and phosphates. In pathological conditions, the presence of albumin and or sugar may be major factors.

Isosthenuria is a condition, in which the specific gravity of urine is fixed and low at 1.010 and does not vary at day and night.

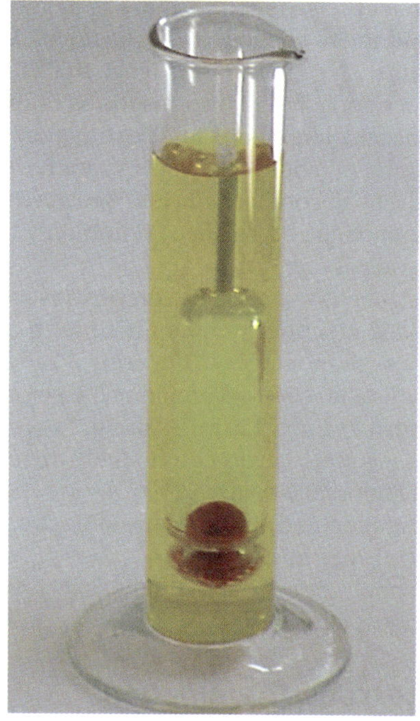

FIGURE 15.1 Urinometer

Estimation of Urine Specific Gravity

The estimation of specific gravity of urine is done by urinometer. It is a weighted cylinder that floats in the urine with the stem reading from 1.000 to 1.060 with divisions of 0.001 to 0.002. Urine is poured into a cylinder or conical glass vessel so that it is nearly full. Urinometer is floated in urine and care is taken to see that it does not touch the sides or the bottom of the container. Reading is taken at the lower meniscus. If the volume of urine is insufficient for measuring the specific gravity, it may be diluted with equal volume of distilled water in 1:2 dilution and then multiply the last two digits of the reading by two to get the correct value (Fig. 15.1).

Corrections in Measurement

Correction for Temperature

Urinometer is calibrated for a certain temperature and this is marked on it at 15° or 20°C. Readings at temperature above or below the temperature of calibration needs to be corrected.

Urine, like other fluids expands as the temperature rises. This lowers the specific gravity. At cold temperature, urine contracts or compresses and this reduces the specific gravity.

To correct a specific gravity reading for temperature, note down the room temperature. Then add 0.001 to the reading, for each three degrees above the temperature for which the urinometer is calibrated.

Subtract 0.001 from the reading for each three degrees if the room temperature is below the temperature of calibration.

Example:

- Room temperature—30°C
- Calibration temperature—15°
- Specific gravity of urine measured 1.011
- Corrected specific gravity = [30–15]0.001/3 + 1.011 = 1.016.

Solids in Urine

It is calculated by multiplying the last two digits of the specific gravity of a 24-hour specimen at 15 degrees by 2.016. This figure is called Long's coefficient. Approximate estimate of the amount of solids in 1.000 mL of urine is thus obtained. Normal in an adult is 60 grams.

High Specific Gravity

High specific gravity is seen in excessive sweating, glycosuria and acute nephrites.

Proteins in Urine

Normally, only a small amount of protein is excreted in urine (30–150 mg/day). If the amount of protein excreted in urine is more than this, it is called proteinuria.

Types of Proteinuria

Accidental: This type of proteinuria originates from the lower part of urinary tract and not the kidney. It may be due to the contamination of urine with blood, pus, vaginal discharge or the bladder.

Functional: This type of proteinuria has its origin in the kidney, but does not have any pathological significance. It is called physiological proteinuria. It is intermittent and sometimes has a relation to the posture of the individual. This type of proteinuria is seen in:

- After excessive exercise, especially if not well-trained.
- After prolonged cold bath.
- After excessive protein ingestion.
- Later stages of pregnancy.
- Sometimes in infants.

The proteinuria related to posture is called orthostatic or postural proteinuria. This type of proteinuria is seen when the person is up and walking about for some time, but not when the person is lying down, so that night and early morning urine specimens does not show proteinuria, but samples during the day show proteinuria.

Renal proteinuria: This is also called pathological proteinuria. The proteins in urine are either because of increased permeability for proteins through glomerular capillaries or through the walls of the tubular capillaries and epithelium or both. It is usually persistent.

It is seen in:

- Nephrotic syndrome.
- Acute glomerulonephritis.
- Chronic glomerulonephritis.
- Inflammatory and degenerative diseases of the kidney.
- Febrile or toxic conditions.
- Chemical poisoning by mercury, arsenic or lead.
- Eclampsia—toxemia of pregnancy.

Nature of protein in urine:

- Albumin
- Globulin
- Mucus/mucin
- Hemoglobin and myoglobin
- Bence-Jone protein

Tests for the presence of proteins in urine:

Heat Coagulation Test

Principle: The test is based on the precipitation of proteins by heat.

Procedure: Urine is taken up to three-fourth of the test tube. The upper part of the test tube is heated keeping the lower part as a control. The appearance of turbidity indicates the presence of proteins. About 2 to 3 drops of 3 percent acetic acid is added to the turbid urine. If the turbidity deepens then it is due to presence of proteins in the urine. If the turbidity disappears, then it is due to phosphates and sulfates.

Interpretation of Results

Negative: No cloudiness.

Trace: Cloudiness just visible.

- 1+: Definite cloud without granular flocculation.
- 2+: Heavy and granular cloud without flocculation.
- 3+: Dense cloud with marked flocculation.
- 4+: Thick, curdy precipitate and coagulum.

Sulfosalicylic Acid Test

Principle: It is based on the coagulation of proteins by addition of acid.

Procedure: 2 mL of urine is taken in a test tube and 2 mL of 20 percent sulphosalicylic acid is added to it. Appearance of cloudiness or turbidity indicates the presence of proteins in the urine.

Results

Negative: No cloudiness.
Trace: Cloudiness just visible against dark background.

- 1+: Dense cloudiness.
- 2+: Cloudiness with granules and definite flocculation.
- 3+: Cloudiness with heavy flocculation.
- 4+: Cloudiness with flocculation and precipitation.

Heller's Test

Principle: Precipitation of proteins by using concentrated nitric acid.

Procedure: 2 mL of concentrated nitric acid is taken in a test tube and urine is layered on top of it. Appearance of a white ring at the junction of two liquids indicates the presence of proteins in urine. This is a very sensitive test for the detection of proteins.

Dip Stick Tests

This method is used in most of the laboratories these days.

Sugar in Urine

Presence of sugar in urine is called milleturia. Presence of glucose in urine is called *glycosuria.* This glycosuria occurs when the blood or the plasma glucose level exceeds.

About 180 to 200 mg/dL. It is possible to have glycosuria with low blood glucose if the renal threshold is low and this condition is called renal glycosuria.

Tests for the presence of sugar in urine:

Benedict's Test

Principle: Copper sulfate is reduced to cuprous oxide by the reducing sugars in urine and the color of the resultant precipitate in the blue reagent allows semi-quantitation of the reaction.

Benedict's reagent: It contains crystalline copper sulfate, anhydrous sodium carbonate and sodium citrate.

Procedure: 5 mL of Benedict's reagent is taken in a test tube and eight drops of urine is added to it. Then it is boiled for 2 to 3 minutes. In presence of sugars, the precipitate will turn green to yellow, orange and red depending on the amount of sugars present.

Results

Negative: No change in color.

1+: Green colored precipitate
2+: Yellow to orange colored precipitate
3+: Orange to red precipitate
4+: Brick red precipitate

Other tests for sugar include Fehling's test and glucose oxidase test.

Conditions in which glycosuria is seen—
Diabetes mellitus.

Ketone Bodies in Urine

Ketone bodies are intermediate products of fat metabolism. The presence of ketone bodies in urine is called ketonuria. The three main ketone bodies are acetone, acetoacetic acid and betahydroxybutyric acid.

Tests for the presence of ketone bodies in urine:

Rothera's Test

Principle: Acetone and diacetic acid react with sodium nitroprusside in presence of alkali to produce a purple color.

Procedure: 5 mL of urine is taken in a test tube and is saturated with ammonium sulfate. 1 crystal of sodium nitroprusside is added to it. Then 0.5 to 1 mL of liquor ammonia is layered on to it. The appearance of purple color indicates the presence of ketone bodies in urine.

Other tests to detect ketone bodies in urine are Gerhardt test and Hart's test.

Conditions in which ketonuria is seen:
- Diabetic ketoacidosis
- Starvation ketoacidosis
- Prolonged febrile states
- Uncontrolled vomiting and diarrhea.

Blood in Urine

Presence of RBCs in urine is called as *hematuria*. Presence of hemoglobin in urine is called as *hemoglobinuria*. To differentiate between the two the sample of urine is centrifuged and the sediment is examined under the microscope. The presence of intact RBCs under the microscope indicates hematuria.

Benzidine Test

Principle: Peroxidase enzyme in hemoglobin or RBC will convert hydrogen peroxide to nascent oxygen, which in acidic medium will oxidize benzidine to give a blue color.

Reagents: Saturated solution of benzidine in glacial acetic acid and hydrogen peroxide.

Procedure: 2 mL of hydrogen peroxide is taken in a test tube, a pinch of benzidine is added to it and heated. 5 mL of urine is added to it and it is layered with freshly prepared glacial acetic acid. Green color turning to blue indicates the presence of blood in urine.

Microscopic Examination of Urine

The urine is taken in a test tube and centrifuged at 1500 rpm for 5 minutes and then are sediment is examined under the microscope. A thin preparation under the cover slip, without any air bubbles is made.

Urinary sediment is divided into:
1. Unorganized sediment.
2. Organized sediment.

Unorganized sediment consists of crystals of various substances present in urine. These crystals vary in different pH.

Crystals found in acidic urine are: Uric acid, urates, calcium oxalate crystals, cystine crystals, leucine, sulfa crystals and tyrosine crystals.

Crystals found in alkaline urine are: Ammonium magnesium phosphates, dicalcium phosphates, calcium carbonate and ammonium biurate crystals.

Organized sediment consists of tubular casts, hyaline casts, granular casts, epithelial cell casts, blood cell casts, pus cell casts, fatty casts and waxy casts.

EXAMINATION OF FECES

Stool specimens are examined to know:
- The presence and the type of parasites.
- Differentiation between bacillary and amebic dysentery and diagnosis of cholera and other diarrheal diseases.
- Presence of occult blood and stool fat by chemical tests to evaluate colorectal cancer, malabsorption, etc.

Collection

Stool sample is collected in a wide mouthed glass or plastic bottle. About 1 to 2 g may be sufficient. It is examined within one hour of collection. The preservative like formal saline can be used.

Macroscopic Examination

- *Quantity:* Bulkier stools are seen with vegetarian diets than meat diets and also in malabsorption syndromes. Patients on antibiotics pass less feces.
- *Consistency and form:* Normally, it is well formed. In constipation, feces is passed as small hard masses. It is fluid or watery in severe diarrhea, dysentery and after purgative use.

  In cholera, stools are copious, thin, very watery, colorless and has white flakes of desquamated epithelium. It is called "rice water stools".

  In malabsorption, stools are pale, bulky, soft and semisolid with froth.

- *Color:* Normally it is light to dark brown due to presence of bile pigments. Bleeding in the intestine makes it reddish. Tarry black stools indicate bleeding in the upper GIT. It is called 'melena'. Stools are clay colored in biliary obstruction.
- *Odor:* The odor of stools is due to the presence of indole and skatole and is more with meat diets. When undigested and unabsorbed fat is present, it causes foul odor.
- *Mucus:* Increased mucus is seen in conditions like colitis. In amebic dysentery both blood and mucus are seen which differentiates it from bacillary dysentery.
- *Parasites:* Number of parasites may be seen in feces. It can be roundworms, hookworms, threadworms (segments or whole worms), larvae and ova.

Microscopic Examination

Preparation of stool specimens for microscopy:

- *Saline preparation:* A little fecal material is taken on a slide with a narrow stick and mixed with a drop of saline. A coverslip is placed on it and examined under micro scope.
- *Iodine preparation:* Here instead of saline a drop of Gram's iodine solution is used. Iodine stains are the nuclear structures of cysts.

Stool Concentration Techniques

When the parasites are scanty in stools, routine microscopic examination may not give positive results. It is, therefore, necessary to concentrate the ova and cysts in the sample.

Floatation Method

In this technique, zinc sulfate solution with a specific gravity of 1.180 is prepared. Both helminth ova and protozoal cysts have a specific gravity less than 1.180. So, they float to the surface while the faecal matter sinks to the bottom.

Sedimentation Method

In this technique, called formalin-ether concentration method, the ova and cysts will appear in the sediment after centrifugation rather than at the surface due to floatation.

Microscopic examination of feces is done by selecting the mucoid and blood stained mucoid part of stool when available and following are detected.

- Cells—pus cells, red blood cells, macrophages, epithelial cells and yeast cells.
- Crystals like Charcot-Leyden crystals, fat globules.
- Parasites—trophozoites and cysts, eggs and larvae.

Chemical Tests on Feces

- *Tests for occult blood*: It is possible to have significant loss of blood in the intestine due to parasites or cancer without finding abnormal color in the feces. To detect occult blood, three types of reagents can be used. They are gum guaiacum, benzidine and orthotolidine. The sensitivity of orthotolidine is greater than the other two.
- *Tests for fat in the stool:* Presence of free fat and its quantitative determination is done. It helps in the accurate diagnosis of steatorrhea or sprue.
- *Tests for stercobilinogen/stercobilin:* It is done to diagnose hemolytic anemia.
- *Tests for reducing substances in the feces:* It is done in lactose intolerance seen in some infants.

Stool Culture

The feces is inoculated onto a various media like MacConkey's agar, desoxycholate citrate agar, etc. incubated at 37°C overnight. The next day, various colonies are found which are examined and subcultured.

SECTION 2

Genetics

CHAPTER 16

Introduction

GENETICS IS THE STUDY OF GENES

Practical Application of Genetics in Nursing

Today, genetics is the branch of medicine which is fast expanding. The basis of every disease is now identified up to the level of genetic mutation. The unraveling of human genome project was an important landmark in the history of genetics. As nursing is a branch closely associated with medicine and patient care, it is mandatory for the nurses to know about the basics of genetics. This knowledge about genetics will enable the nurses to deliver more rational healthcare to their patients.

IMPACT OF GENETIC CONDITION ON FAMILIES

Genetics deals with the identification of the mutation leading to a particular disease. These genetic mutations have a particular pattern of inheritance. Many of the genetic diseases run in families. The knowledge about such genetic diseases and their pattern of inheritance will allow for genetic mapping and genetic counseling of prospective parents, thus avoiding unnecessary mental trauma. *See* Figures 16.4 to 16.6 for the schematic representation of dominant inheritance pattern, recessive inheritance pattern and X-linked inheritance pattern respectively.

REVIEW OF CELLULAR DIVISION

Every living cell divides. There are two types of cell division:

Mitosis

Mitosis is the division of a single cell with both the daughter cells having same genetic material as the parent cell. This type of cell division is seen in cell growth, differentiation and repair. The parent cell has 46 chromosomes (23 pairs). Each of the daughter cells will have the same number of chromosomes, that is, 46 chromosomes and hence are called diploid. Mitosis occurs in all the cells of the body except ova and sperms (Fig. 16.1).

Meiosis

Meiosis is a type of cell division, where each daughter cell will have half the number of chromosomes of the parent cell. So, each daughter cell will have 23 chromosomes in contrast to the 46 chromosomes of the parent cell. This type of cell division occurs in ova and sperms. As the daughter cell has only one copy of each chromosome, these are called haploid. This is also called reduction division (Fig. 16.2).

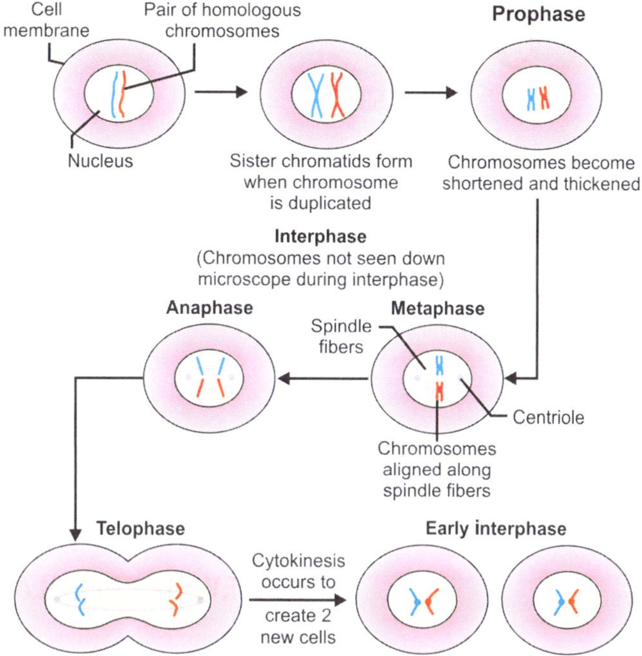

FIGURE 16.1 Mitosis

Both the types of cell divisions have four phases namely, *Prophase, Metaphase, Anaphase* and *Telophase*. In meiosis, as it is reduction division, there are two sets of all four stages.

CHARACTERISTICS AND STRUCTURE OF GENES

Genes are the units of heredity and are composed of parts of specific DNA molecules. DNA is the chemical component of chromosomes which is seen in all nucleated cells. The genes are arranged in linear series within the chromosomes.

Structure of DNA

The double helical model of DNA was proposed by Watson and Crick in 1953. According to this model, the DNA has two strands and each strand has four different types of nucleic acids namely adenine (A), guanine (G), cytosine (C) and thymidine (T). The DNA is unique as adenine always pairs with thymidine (A → T) and guanine always pairs with cytosine (G → C). The purine bases are A and G. The pyrimidine bases are C and T. The two strands of DNA are linked by hydrogen bonds. There are two hydrogen bonds between A and T and three hydrogen bonds between C and G (Fig. 16.3).

Karyotyping: It is the diagrammatic representation of the chromosomes of an individual. The cells are arrested in the metaphase and a picture of the chromosomal complement is taken.

Sex chromatin: It is the inactivated X-ray chromosome seen in the females. This is normally seen in the buccal smear cells as a dark condensed body and is referred to as the "Barr body". The Barr body helps to identify the gender as female.

CHROMOSOMAL ABERRATION

An abnormality in either the number or the structure of the chromosome is called as

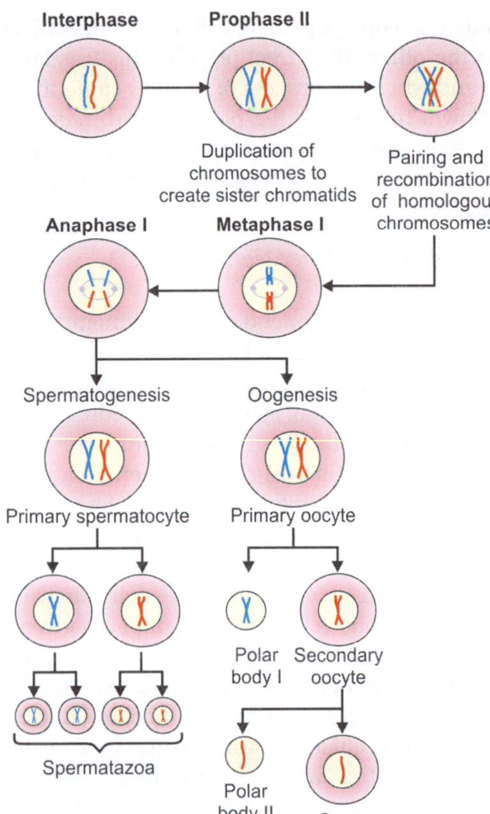

FIGURE 16.2 Meiosis

chromosomal aberration. These aberrations usually result from an error in the cell division during mitosis/meiosis.

Numerical Chromosomal Aberration

When a chromosome is missing from a pair, it is called *monosomy*, e.g. Turner syndrome, where there is one X chromosome missing with XO chromosomal complement. When an extra chromosome is seen in a pair, it is called *trisomy*, e.g. trisomy 21 is (Down syndrome), trisomy 13 (Patau syndrome) and trisomy 18 (Edwards syndrome).

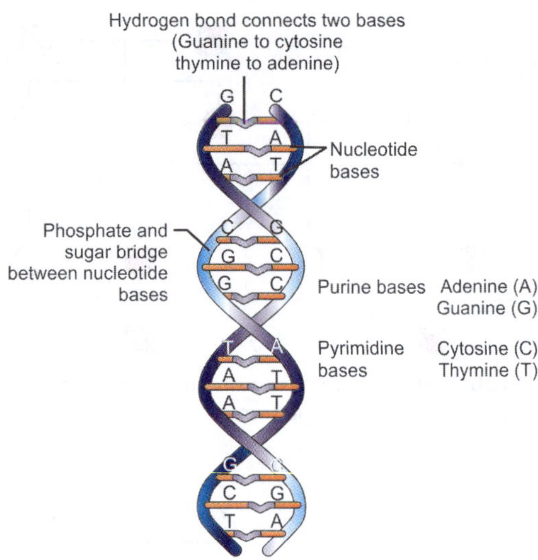

FIGURE 16.3 Structure of DNA

Structural Chromosomal Aberration

When the structure of the chromosome is altered, structural aberrations results. There are different types, namely:

- Deletion
- Duplication
- Translocation
- Inversion
- Isochromosome.

Factors affecting chromosomal aberrations:

- Genetic factors
- Radiation
- Environmental factors.

Mendelian Theory of Inheritance

Sir Gregor John Mendel was the first person to put forward a hypothesis regarding the transmission of hereditary characters from the parent to the children.

Mendel's Laws

Mendel summarized his findings in two laws; the Law of Segregation and the Law of Independent Assortment.

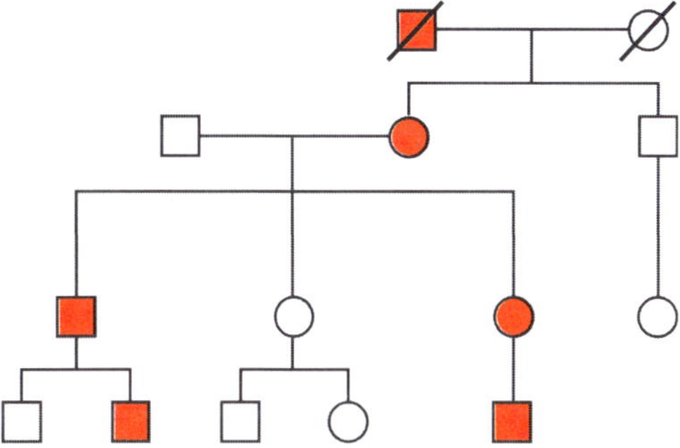

FIGURE 16.4 Features of a dominant inheritance pattern

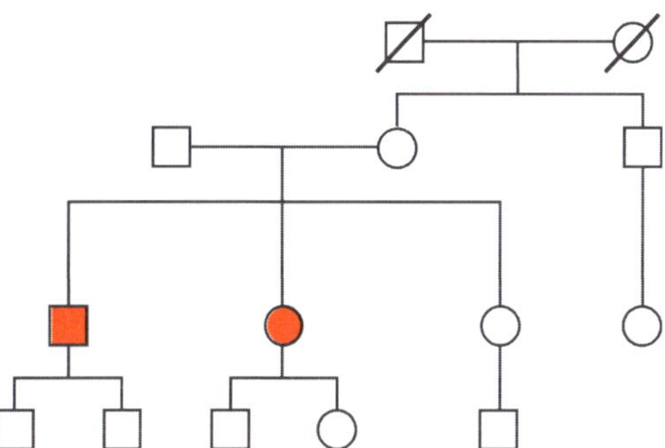

FIGURE 16.5 Features of a recessive inheritance pattern

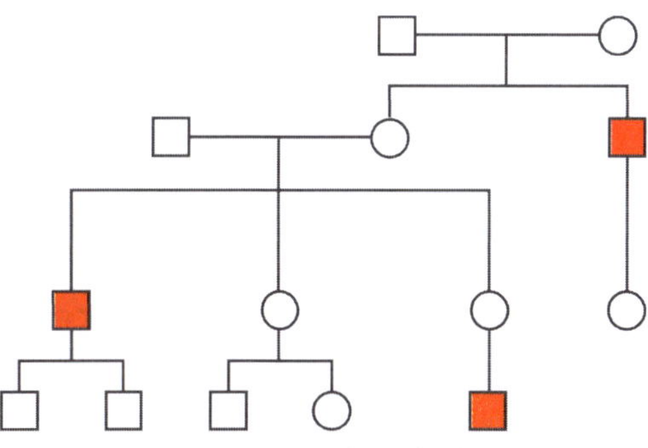

FIGURE 16.6 Features of X-linked inheritance pattern

Law of Segregation (The "First Law")

The Law of Segregation states that when any individual produces gametes, the copies of a gene separate, so that each gamete receives only one copy. A gamete will receive one allele or the other. The direct proof of this was later found when the process of meiosis came to be known. In meiosis, the paternal and maternal chromosomes get separated and the alleles with the characters are segregated into two different gametes.

Law of Independent Assortment (The "Second Law")

The Law of Independent Assortment, also known as "Inheritance Law", states that alleles of different genes assort independently of one another during gamete formation. While Mendel's experiments with mixing one trait always resulted in a 3:1 ratio between dominant and recessive phenotypes, his experiments with mixing two traits (dihybrid cross) showed 9:3:3:1 ratios. Mendel concluded that different traits are inherited independently of each other, so that there is no relation, for example, between a cat's color and tail length. This is actually only true for genes that are not linked to each other.

Independent assortment occurs during meiosis I in eukaryotic organisms, specifically metaphase I of meiosis, to produce a gamete with a mixture of the organism's maternal and paternal chromosomes. Along with chromosomal crossover, this process aids in increasing genetic diversity by producing novel genetic combinations.

Among the 46 chromosomes in a normal diploid human cell, half are maternally-derived (from the mother's egg) and half are paternally-derived (from the father's sperm). This occurs as sexual reproduction involves the fusion of two haploid gametes (the egg and sperm) to produce a new organism having the full complement of chromosomes. During gametogenesis, the production of new gametes by an adult—the normal complement of 46 chromosomes needs to be halved to 23 to ensure that the resulting haploid gamete can join with another gamete to produce a diploid organism. An error in the number of chromosomes, such as those caused by a diploid gamete joining with a haploid gamete, is termed aneuploidy.

In independent assortment, the chromosomes that end up in a newly-formed gamete are randomly sorted from all possible combinations of maternal and paternal chromosomes. Because gametes end up with a random mix instead of a pre-defined "set" from either parent, gametes are, therefore considered assorted independently. As such, the gamete can end up with any combination of paternal or maternal chromosomes. Any of the possible combinations of gametes formed from maternal and paternal chromosomes will occur with equal frequency. For human gametes, with 23 pairs of chromosomes, the number of possibilities is 223 or 8,388,608 possible combinations. The gametes will normally end up with 23 chromosomes, but the origin of any particular one will be randomly selected from paternal or maternal chromosomes. This contributes to the genetic variability of progeny.

CHAPTER 17

Maternal, Prenatal and Genetic Influences on Development of Defects and Diseases

CONDITIONS AFFECTING THE MOTHER: GENETIC AND INFECTIONS

Skeletal Dysplasia

There are a large number of different types of skeletal dysplasia. This is a term used to describe a number of conditions in which the skeleton forms in an unusual way, causing bony deformity. The genetic code for the formation of the skeleton is faulty. A child may be at risk of skeletal dysplasia if either parent is affected, but if the mother is affected then preconceptual care is useful, as the condition of the pelvis and spine can be assessed prior to pregnancy. The bony deformity may affect the lie of the fetus in the third trimester, and may make passage of the fetus through the birth canal difficult in labor.

A similar situation may occur if the mother has a neural tube defect.

Maternal Diabetes

Maternal diabetes is known to affect the growth and development of the fetus. In poorly controlled diabetic mothers, there is an increase in the rate of spontaneous abortions. Intrauterine growth retardation occurs more frequently in the babies of diabetic mothers.

Rather than being a direct effect of abnormal glucose levels, it is more likely to be due to a complex interaction between glucose levels, ketone bodies and decreased availability of insulin.

Macrosomia of the fetus may also occur. Congenital malformations occur significantly more frequently in infants of diabetic mothers. The teratogenic effects seem to occur very early in the pregnancy (up to the seventh week). For this reason, preconceptual counseling of diabetic mothers is helpful. Strict blood control of blood glucose levels has been shown to decrease the rate of congenital malformations.

CONNECTIVE TISSUE DISORDERS (MARFAN SYNDROME AND EHLERS-DANLOS SYNDROME)

Marfan syndrome is a dominant condition that affects a number of different body systems. The genetic defect adversely affects the development of connective tissue, namely collagen. Marfan syndrome causes tall stature, hypermobility of the joints, cardiovascular abnormalities, aortic root dilatation and aortic aneurysm, and dislocated lenses. Owing to the joint laxity and stature, serious back pain in pregnancy may become a problem. The mother with Marfan syndrome who has an existing cardiovascular abnormality should be under the care of a

cardiologist, who should be made aware of the pregnancy.

There are two main issues concerned with the management of pregnancy in these cases. First, the woman should have a baseline cardiac assessment if the condition is one in which cardiac complications can occur. Second, tissue friability should be assessed as the stretching of the uterine tissue in pregnancy may lead to uterine rupture, and if this is a significant risk the couple should be aware of this before pregnancy occurs.

The term Ehlers-Danlos syndrome (EDS) refers to a group of disorders of connective tissue. Hyperextensibility of skin, increased mobility of joints and tissue fragility are common features. Women with this condition may be at higher risk of spontaneous abortion and stillbirth. It is thought that collagen in the chorionic membranes is affected by the condition, making premature rupture of membranes more likely. Because of the fragility of vessel walls, these women will also be at increased risk of hemorrhage antenatally and during labor.

Epilepsy

Epilepsy is a condition, in which the offspring of a person with epilepsy has a greater chance than others in the general population of developing the condition. However, it is not inherited as a single gene disorder. If a mother has epilepsy, there is a danger of fetal hypoxia during a fit, and, therefore, the aim of treatment must be to avoid seizures during the pregnancy. The prospective mother should be advised to try and stabilize the epilepsy before conception. However, the use of drug therapy is not without additional risk to the fetus, as many anticonvulsants are known to cause serious congenital abnormalities.

Women who are taking anticonvulsants are in the group considered to be at increased risk of having a child with a Neural Tube Defect (NTD) and should therefore, be prescribed the higher dose folic acid (5 mg daily), to be taken preconceptually for at least 2 months and for the first 3 months of pregnancy.

Maternal Phenylketonuria

Phenylketonuria (PKU) is a recessive condition, in which the biochemical pathway involved in the metabolism of phenylalanine is disturbed, causing increased phenylalanine levels in the affected person. The accumulation of phenylalanine in the body results in mental retardation; however, the use of a low phenylalanine diet during infancy, childhood and adolescence will dramatically reduce the risk of mental retardation.

It has been shown that during pregnancy high maternal levels of phenylalanine have adverse effects on the fetus, causing microcephaly, mental retardation, dysmorphic features and congenital heart disease.

It is, therefore, strongly advised that women are encouraged to remain on a low phenylalanine diet, to maintain a serum phenylalanine level of 120 to 360 μmol/L until they have completed their families, to reduce the risk to their offspring.

Cystic Fibrosis

Cystic fibrosis (CF) is a common recessive condition. The gene mutation causes a disturbance of chloride, sodium and water ratios in secretions, resulting primarily in respiratory infections, reduced lung function, and reduced pancreatic function.

Where the mother's lung function is normal, the CF does not appear to confer significantly higher risks to mother or fetus, however, where there is impaired function, there is a greater risk of prematurity for the fetus, and therapeutic abortion may be considered to preserve the mother's health. Mothers with CF are prone to develop diabetes and this should be borne in mind when caring for such women. It is important that the mother should be under the care of a respiratory specialist for monitoring at least monthly during the pregnancy.

Hemoglobinopathy

Thalassemia major: For women with thalassemia, a protocol will be used for

treatment with a series of blood transfusions. Iron chelation therapy (desferrioxamine) will also usually be administered to maintain stable serum ferritin levels. Cardiac problems, diabetes and hepatitis C may complicate the pregnancies of women with thalassemia major. Cardiac, hepatic and endocrine function should be monitored during pregnancy and in the postpartum period.

Sickle cell disease: Mothers with sickle cell disease are at increased risk of spontaneous abortion and stillbirth. Severe anemia in pregnancy is treated with blood transfusion.

CONGENITAL HEART DISEASE

A woman with heart disease due to a chromosome 22q microdeletion may have learning difficulties and problems with immunity. Prophylactic antibiotics are often considered during labor. While vaginal delivery is recommended for many conditions, a cesarean section may be the best option in a woman who is already cyanosed and who is being delivered prematurely, and for those women with Marfan syndrome.

In some cases, a congenital heart defect may be so severe that pregnancy is contraindicated and termination of pregnancy to preserve the life of the mother may be advised by a cardiologist.

Certain maternal infections may be transmitted to the infant. Transmission may occur *in utero*, at the time of delivery or, in the case of HIV, during breastfeeding and may be the cause of congenital anomaly and/ or fetal or perinatal infection. Some of them are asymptomatic bacteriuria, chickenpox, *Chlamydia*, group B streptococci, hepatitis B, herpes simplex, HIV, *Mycoplasma*, rubella, syphilis, thrush, toxoplasmosis, *Trichomonas* and many more.

CONSANGUINITY

Consanguineous marriages are those between close relatives, e.g. between cousins. Parental consanguinity is often associated with genetic disorders and congenital malformations in their offsprings. They are at increased risk of having a child with a recessive condition, as both parents could carry the same faulty gene, inherited from the common grandparent or great grandparent. Increased homozygosity is seen which leads to genetic anomalies. Many malformations caused by inheritance in consanguineous marriages are twice as common as in non-consanguineous marriages. The children of second cousins will be at less risk of a recessive condition. The common disorders are psychomotor retardation, mental retardation, metabolic disorders like phenylketonuria, blindness, seizures, etc.

Atopy

Atopy is a term coined by Coca and Cooke in 1923. It refers to a predisposition to develop localized immediate hypersensitivity reactions to a variety of inhaled and ingested allergens. Atopic individuals have higher serum IgE levels and more Interleukin-4 (IL-4) producing T-Helper 2 cells. In 50 percent of the atopic individuals, a positive history of allergy is seen. Many studies have revealed a linkage to several gene loci. Candidate genes have been mapped to 5q31 where genes for the cytokines IL-3, IL-4, IL-5, IL-9, IL-13 and GM-CSF (Granulocyte-macrophage colony stimulating factor) are located giving an idea that these cytokines are involved in the reactions. Linkage has also been noted to 6p, close to HLA complex.

Prenatal Nutrition and Food Allergies

Diet and nutrition during gestation and early infancy is an important determinant of the development of allergy in children. Allergic diseases have emerged as a common cause of illness and mortality in particularly high-risk infants. Allergy to certain foodstuffs can produce a severe anaphylactic reaction. The most well-known example of this type of allergen is peanut,

and death may occur in sensitized individuals as a result of ingesting even minute quantities of peanut or peanut oil in food. There is evidence that in families with a history of allergy, infants may be sensitized to certain allergens while still *in utero*. Prevention of allergy can be aimed at, by exclusive breastfeeding, delayed introduction of allergenic foods to the baby and avoidance of allergenic foods by mother during gestation.

Maternal Age

Advanced maternal age refers to women who are more than 35 years of age at the time of delivery. Prenatal testing for chromosomal abnormalities is to be done in women of this age group.

Fertility in women gradually decreases from early thirties. Women in their late thirties and forties have increased risk of developing gestational diabetes and hypertension during pregnancy. Down's syndrome and other chromosomal disorders are very common in offsprings of women of advanced age. Meiotic nondisjunction is more likely to happen in older women. A woman with advanced age should, therefore, consult a health care provider before planning to conceive. Amniocentesis is a definite indication where a small amount of amniotic fluid from the amniotic sac surrounding the fetus is removed between 15 and 18 weeks of gestation and is used for genetic analysis. It is also important to know that many of the risks associated with these women can be managed with good prenatal care.

Maternal Drug Therapy

Phocomelia, a congenital disorder involving limbs (short or absent long bones) was seen in many newborn babies in the early 1960s. It was connected with prenatal exposure to the drug *thalidomide* used to treat morning sickness in pregnancy. Therefore, pregnant women must be monitored by physician for any kind of drug.

Teratology

Teratology is the study of abnormalities of physiological development. Teratogen is an agent which causes abnormality in the fetus on exposure during pregnancy. Birth defects are known to occur in 3 to 5 percent of all newborns. They are one of the leading causes of infant mortality. After the thalidomide disaster of the 1960s, it became apparent and more accepted that the developing embryo could be highly vulnerable to certain environmental agents that have negligible or nontoxic effects to adult individuals.

Wilson's Six Principles

Along with this, new awareness of the *in utero* vulnerability of the developing mammalian embryo came the development and refinement of *The Six Principles of Teratology*, which are still applied today. These principles of teratology were put forth by Jim Wilson in 1959 and in his monograph 'Environment and Birth Defects.' These principles guide the study and understanding of teratogenic agents and their effects on developing organisms:

- Susceptibility to teratogenesis depends on the genotype of the conceptus and the manner in which this interacts with adverse environmental factors.
- Susceptibility to teratogenesis varies with the developmental stage at the time of exposure to an adverse influence. There are critical periods of susceptibility to agents and organ systems affected by these agents.
- Teratogenic agents act in specific ways on developing cells and tissues to initiate sequences of abnormal developmental events.
- The access of adverse influences to developing tissues depends on the nature of the influence. Several factors affect the ability of a teratogen to contact a developing conceptus, such as the nature of the agent itself, route and degree of maternal

exposure, rate of placental transfer and systemic absorption, and composition of the maternal and embryonic/fetal genotypes.
- There are four manifestations of deviant development (death, malformation, growth retardation and functional defect).
- Manifestations of deviant development increase in frequency and degree as dosage increases from the no observable adverse effect level (NOAEL) to a dose producing 100% lethality (LD100).

Understanding how a teratogen causes its effect is not only important in preventing congenital abnormalities but also has the potential for developing new therapeutic drugs safe for use with pregnant women.

Teratogenic Agents

A wide range of different chemicals and environmental factors are suspected or are known to be teratogenic in humans. A selected few include:

Ionizing radiation: Atomic weapons, radioiodine, radiation therapy.

Infections: Cytomegalovirus, herpes virus, parvovirus B-19, rubella virus (German measles), syphilis, toxoplasmosis, Venezuelan equine encephalitis virus. Several infections which a mother can contact during pregnancy called TORCH (toxoplasma, rubella) infections can also be teratogenic.

Metabolic imbalance: Alcoholism, endemic cretinism, diabetes, folic acid deficiency, iodine deficiency, hyperthermia, phenylketonuria, rheumatic disease and congenital heart block, virilizing tumors.

Drugs and environmental chemicals: Alcohol, 13-cis-retinoic acid, isotretinoin, temazepam, nitrazepam, nimetazepam, aminopterin, androgenic hormones, busulfan, captopril, enalapril, chlorobiphenyls (PCBs), dioxin, coumarin, cyclophosphamide, diethylstilbestrol, diphenylhydantoin (phenytoin, dilantin, epanutin), ethanol, ethidium bromide, etretinate, hexachlorobenzene hexachlorophene, lithium, methimazole, organic mercury, penicillamine, tetracyclines, thalidomide, trimethadione, uranium, methoxyethyl ethers, flusilazole, valproic acid, and many more.

Teratogenic Outcomes

Exposure to teratogens can result in a wide range of structural abnormalities, such as cleft lip, cleft palate, dysmelia, anencephaly, ventricular septal defect. Exposure to a single agent can produce various abnormalities depending on the stage of development it occurs. Specific birth defects are not characteristic of any single agent.

Prenatal Testing and Diagnosis

Prenatal testing is testing for diseases or conditions in a fetus or embryo before it is born. The aim is to detect birth defects, such as neural tube defects, Down syndrome, chromosomal abnormalities, genetic diseases and other conditions, such as spina bifida, cleft palate, Tay-Sachs disease, sickle cell anemia, thalassemia, cystic fibrosis, and fragile X syndrome. Common testing procedures include amniocentesis, sonograms, nuchal translucency ultrasound, serum marker testing, or genetic screening. Diagnostic prenatal testing can be by invasive or non-invasive methods.

Noninvasive Methods

- Examination of the woman's uterus from outside the body
- Ultrasound detection-scans from 7 weeks to confirm pregnancy dates and look for twins. The specialized nuchal scan at 11 to 13 weeks may be used to identify higher risks of Down's syndrome. Later morphology scans from 18 weeks may check for any abnormal development
- Listening to the fetal heartbeat
- External fetal monitoring, often known as a nonstress test.

Less Invasive Methods

- Second trimester maternal serum screening (AFP screening, triple screen, quad screen, or penta screen) can check levels of alpha fetoprotein, β-hCG, inhibin-A, estriol, and h-hCG (hyperglycosolated hCG) in the woman's serum.
- First trimester maternal serum screening can check levels of free β-hCG, PAPP-A, intact or beta hCG, inhibin-A, or h-hCG in the woman's serum, and combine these with the measurement of nuchal translucency (NT). Some institutions also look for the presence of a fetal nasal bone on the ultrasound.
- Integrated, sequential, and contingent screening tests use serum samples from both first and second trimester, as well as the nuchal translucency measurement to calculate risks. With integrated screening, a report is only produced after both samples have been analyzed. With sequential screening, a first report is produced after the first trimester sample has been submitted, and a final report after the second sample. With contingent screening, patients at very high or very low risks will get reports after the first trimester sample has been submitted. Only patients with moderate risk will be asked to submit a second trimester sample, after which they will receive a report combining information from both serum samples and the NT measurement.
- *Detection of fetal blood cells in maternal blood*: With this technique, it is technically possible to obtain a sample of fetal DNA using blood cells from the fetus that have made their way into the woman's bloodstream. Tests such as, Baby Gender Mentor, allegedly use this method to determine the sex of a fetus as early as six weeks into a pregnancy. Recent developments have also allowed such testing to be used to detect fetal aneuploidy. However, fetal blood cells in maternal blood are extremely rare and very fragile, making it very hard to handle and analyze them. Several companies continue to develop technologies that may someday offer a new way to screen or even diagnose chromosomal abnormalities.
- *Preimplantation genetic diagnosis (PGD)*: During *in vitro fertilization* (IVF) procedures, it is possible to sample cells from human embryos priors to the implantation.

More Invasive Methods

- *Chorionic villus sampling:* Involves getting a sample of the chorionic villus and testing it. This can be done earlier than amniocentesis, but may have a higher risk of miscarriage, estimated at 1 percent.
- *Amniocentesis:* This can be done once enough amniotic fluid has developed to sample. Cells from the fetus will be floating in this fluid, and can be separated and tested. Miscarriage risk of amniocentesis is commonly quoted as 0.5 percent (1:200).
- *Embryoscopy and fetoscopy:* Though rarely done, these involve putting a probe into a women's uterus to observe (with a video camera), or to sample blood or tissue from the embryo or fetus.
- *Fetal blood sampling:* Also known as cordocentesis, this procedure tests for chromosomal defects and other problems. For this test, blood is taken from a vein in the umbilical cord. Fetal blood sampling usually is used when the results of amniocentesis, chorionic villus sampling, or ultrasound are unclear. The test results may take a week or more to complete.

The following are some reasons why a patient might consider her risk of birth defects already to be high and should go straight for invasive testing:

- Women over the age of 35
- Women who have previously had premature babies or babies with a birth defect, especially heart or genetic problems
- Women who have high blood pressure, lupus, diabetes, asthma, or epilepsy
- Women who have family histories or ethnic backgrounds prone to genetic disorders, or whose partners have these

- Women who are pregnant with multiples
- Women who have previously had miscarriages.

INFERTILITY

Number of genetic conditions is known to cause subfertility or infertility. These include conditions related to imbalance of the sex chromosomes such as Turner syndrome in the female (45, X), and Klinefelter syndrome in the male (47, XXY). Female carriers of Fragile X may experience premature ovarian failure, and males with cystic fibrosis may have oligospermia or complete absence of the vas deferens. Such couples are to be offered a referral to an *assisted reproduction unit* for assessment.

Male infertility is often the result of a gene mutation on the Y chromosome. Previously men who carried this mutation would not have had the chance of passing it on to their offspring, but with the new methods they are able to have children and thus produce sons who are similarly infertile. If a mother presents having already had several miscarriages, a balanced chromosome translocation in one of the parents should be suspected. Chromosome studies for both parents should be offered.

Spontaneous Abortion (Miscarriage)

Spontaneous abortion is thought to occur in approximately 10 to 15 percent of confirmed pregnancies. Women with a history of miscarriage are less likely to carry subsequent pregnancies to term. There are many causes of spontaneous abortion, these include:

- Anatomical abnormality (e.g. bicornuate uterus)
- Infection (e.g. herpes, cytomegalovirus or rubella)
- Maternal hormonal imbalance (e.g. progesterone deficiency)
- Endocrine dysfunction in the mother (e.g. poorly controlled diabetes)
- Maternal immunological abnormality (e.g. systemic lupus erythematosus).

However, an unbalanced chromosome arrangement in the fetus is believed to be the cause of up to 50 percent of spontaneous abortions. In any pregnancy, there is a risk that the fetus will have an unbalanced chromosome arrangement. The chromosomal imbalance may occur sporadically, or more infrequently it is inherited from a parent with a chromosome translocation. Because most cases of chromosomal imbalance in a fetus occur sporadically, the parents have a low risk of the same problem occurring for a second time. Thus, a mother who has conceived one child with a chromosomal abnormality will usually have a less than one percent chance of having another child with that condition.

A balanced translocation as a cause of spontaneous abortion is usually not suspected until there has been at least two, but usually three, pregnancies lost in this way. After recurrent abortion, it is good to investigate the chromosome patterns of both parents. If one of the parents has a balanced translocation or rearrangement, there will normally be at least a 50 percent chance that in each pregnancy the fetus will inherit a balanced chromosome arrangement and, therefore, will develop normally.

Neural Tube Defects and the Role of Folic Acid in Lowering the Risks

The neural tube lies along the back of a developing embryo and becomes the brain and spinal cord. Neural tube defects are abnormalities of the embryo's brain and spinal cord. Folic acid supplements can prevent neural tube defects (NTD) and other malformations. Women who take folic acid vitamin supplements before and during early pregnancy are less likely to have babies with neural tube defects than women who do not take folic acid. NTD malformations include spina bifida (open spine); meningomyeloceles, myeloceles; anencephaly (open skull); encephalocele (gap in the skull) and other anomalies.

Enough folic acid cannot be obtained by diet alone. Over 70 percent of NTD and

other birth defects can be prevented by taking 4 mg of folic acid each day prior to conception and in the first three months of pregnancy. All women capable of pregnancy should take a daily vitamin supplement that contains 0.4 to 0.8 mg of folic acid, because most pregnancies are unexpected. Starting to take folic acid only when pregnant is too late.

Down Syndrome (Trisomy 21)

Down syndrome is the most common of the chromosomal disorders and is a major cause of mental retardation. Approximately, 95 percent of the affected individuals have trisomy 21, so their chromosome count is 47. The major cause is meiotic nondisjunction.

Maternal age has a very strong influence in Down syndrome. Incidence increases in mothers over 35 years of age. The diagnostic clinical features of this syndrome are flat facial profile, oblique palpebral fissures and epicanthic folds. The IQ of the 80 percent of the affected individuals is seen in between 25 and 50. Approximately, 40 percent have congenital heart diseases like endocardial cushion defects, ostium primum, atrial septal defect, arterio-venous malformation and ventricular septal defect. Children with trisomy 21 have a 10 to 20 fold increased risk of developing acute leukemia. Patients with trisomy 21 older than 40 years of age develop Alzheimer disease, a degenerative disorder of brain. There is increased incidence of infections in these patients.

Antenatal Screening for Down Syndrome

Amniocentesis is usually offered to all women who will be over a certain age at the birth of the baby, normally 35 or 37. Various screening methods involving biochemical testing of the mother's blood and ultrasound scanning have been developed in an attempt to identify individual women whose pregnancy may be at increased risk. These include:

First Trimester

- Nuchal translucency measurement by ultrasound
- Double test on maternal serum, pregnancy-associated plasma protein A (PAPP-A) and human chorionic gonadotropin (hCG)
- Combined nuchal translucency and double test.

Second Trimester

- Double test on maternal serum, alpha-fetoprotein (AFP) and hCG
- Triple test on maternal serum, AFP, hCG and unconjugated estriol (uE3)
- Quadruple test on maternal serum, AFP, hCG, uE3, inhibin A.

  The *integrated test* involves testing in both first and second trimester:
  - Nuchal translucency and PAPP-A in first trimester
  - Quadruple test in second trimester.

However, these tests only provide an estimation of the chance the fetus will have Down syndrome, rather than a definitive result. If the risk is greater than one in 250 the mother is usually offered a test to check the karyotype of the fetus.

New techniques for extracting fetal cells from a maternal blood sample are being developed.

CHAPTER 18

Genetic Testing in Neonates and Children

Screening the neonates and children is a good practice in today's medical technology. Now, it is possible to diagnose many genetic diseases *in utero*. Once diagnosed, these anomalies can be minimized before there are irreversible deleterious effects on the fetus.

Neonatal screening is done by testing blood sample of the newborn for certain fatal diseases. These diseases include homocystinuria, phenylketonuria, hypothyroidism and galactosemia. These tests ensure minimal risk to the neonate and maximal long time benefits. The early detection of such disorders will positively have an impact on the treatment of such babies.

SCREENING FOR CONGENITAL ABNORMALITIES

A congenital anomaly (congenital abnormality, congenital malformation, birth defect) is a condition, which is present at the time of birth, which varies from the standard presentation.

Types

A limb anomaly is called a dysmelia. These include all forms of limb anomalies, such as amelia, ectrodactyly, phocomelia, polymelia, polydactyly, syndactyly, polysyndactyly, oligodactyly, brachydactyly, achondroplasia, congenital aplasia or hypoplasia, amniotic band syndrome, and cleidocranial dysostosis.

Congenital anomalies of the heart include patent ductus arteriosus, atrial septal defect, ventricular septal defect, and tetralogy of Fallot.

Congenital anomalies of the nervous system include neural tube defects, such as spina bifida, meningocele, meningomyelocele, encephalocele and anencephaly. Other congenital anomalies of the nervous system include the Arnold-Chiari malformation, the Dandy-Walker malformation, hydrocephalus, microencephaly, megencephaly, lissencephaly, polymicrogyria, holoprosencephaly, and agenesis of the corpus callosum.

Congenital anomalies of the gastrointestinal system include numerous forms of stenosis and atresia, and imperforate anus.

The cause of 40 to 60 percent of congenital anomalies in humans is unknown. These are referred to as sporadic. Genetic causes of congenital anomalies include inheritance of abnormal genes from the parents, as well as new mutations in one of the germ cells that gave rise to the fetus. Environmental causes of congenital anomalies are referred to as teratogenic.

DEVELOPMENTAL DELAY

Developmental delay is defined as a delay in reaching the normal milestones within

the normal age range for each milestone, for example, failure to walk before the age of 18 months. Development tasks are usually divided into categories, related to motor tasks, speech and cognition. If delay is suspected, the child's development may be assessed formally using a recognized developmental test. This type of tool requires the child to complete a series of tasks; each designed to assess a different aspect of development, in the motor, speech or cognitive sphere. The tasks are assigned different points, and the number of points compared with that expected for the child's age.

Example of developmental assessment tool: Locomotor skills involving the use of stairs would be judged, with a child who crawls upstairs attaining 1 point, and one who is able to run upstairs being allocated 6 points.

DYSMORPHISM

Dysmorphism is defined as an unusual pattern of physical features. An abnormal gene or chromosome structure often alters the physical features in that child. Although these unusual characteristics are themselves usually completely benign, they provide clues as to the gene or chromosome abnormality in that child. Children who share the same genetic abnormality will share common characteristics, and although unrelated, may look very similar to one another. The well-known example of children, who have the same chromosome abnormality looking similar, is Down syndrome. It is easy to identify a person with Down syndrome, because of the similar facial and body characteristics of those who have inherited an additional chromosome 21. Children with Down syndrome will also inherit some particular physical features that identify them as belonging to their family.

Common Dysmorphic Features

Head

- Microcephaly—head size below 3rd centile
- Macrocephaly—head size above 97th centile
- Hydrocephaly—head size increased, due to excess fluid in ventricles
- Delayed closure of fontanelles
- Flat or prominent occiput
- Craniosynostosis—abnormal joining of the bones of the skull, resulting in abnormal head shape.

Hair

- Abnormally thick or thin hair
- Double crown
- Sparse hair.

Eyes

- Hypotelorism—short space between eyes
- Hypertelorism—long space between eyes
- Slanting palpebral fissures (eye opening)
- Epicanthic folds—folds of skin at inner canthus of the eye
- Prominent eyes
- Microphthalmia (small eye) or anophthalmia (absence of eye)
- Blue sclera
- Coloboma—'gap' in iris
- Cataract.

Mouth

- Clefting of lips or palate
- Prominent lips
- Lip pits
- Macroglossia
- Hypoplasia of teeth enamel
- Small or abnormally shapen teeth
- Irregular placement of teeth.

Ears

- Malformation of auricles
- Low-set ears
- Preauricular tags or pits.

Hands/feet

- Brachydactyly
- Clinodactyly
- Hypoplasia of thumb or fingers

- Hypoplasia of metacarpals
- Polydactyly
- Syndactyly
- Broad thumb or toe.

Genitalia

- Hypospadius
- Undescended testes
- Unusually large or small penis/testes
- Hypoplasia of labia majora
- Vaginal atresia.

Stature

- Stature above 97th or below 3rd centile for age
- Disproportion between trunk and limbs.

Skin

- Excessive or inadequate sweating
- Altered skin pigmentation
- Hemangiomata
- Thick or ichthyotic skin.

Spine

- Neural tube defect
- Scoliosis
- Kyphosis.

CNS

- Hypertonicity
- Hypotonicity.

CHAPTER 19

Genetic Conditions of Adolescents and Adults

CANCER GENETICS: FAMILIAL CANCER

In the majority of cases, cancer occurs as a sporadic event, due to changes in the genes in a particular cell (somatic change). If a person presents with a family history of cancer, we need to work out if a number of cancers have occurred coincidentally in the family, or if there is a family gene mutation being inherited by some family members. Although there are a number of rare cancer syndromes, such as Von Hippel-Lindau disease, in general the majority of familial cancers will be connected with colorectal cancer or breast/ovarian cancer.

The function of some genes is to help prevent the growth of cancers and these are called *tumor suppressor genes*. Whenever new cells are produced in the body to replace dead or damaged cells, the tumor suppressor gene limits the number of new cells, thus preventing overgrowth of the tissue. If the particular sequence of these genes is correct, then the protective action of the genes is intact. However, the genetic material is recopied over and over again during the person's lifetime, as new cells are made. Each time the gene is copied, there is the potential for a mistake to be made. If one copy of the gene becomes faulty, then the person will usually develop a tumor.

Knudson first described the *two-hit hypothesis* in development of cancer in retinoblastoma, and the hypothesis helps us to make sense of what occurs in familial cancer. If a person is born with one faulty copy of a gene, then they are likely to develop cancer at a younger age, because they only need one more accidental fault in the gene to occur to make both copies faulty. Figure 19.1 shows the schematic representation of two hit/Knudson's hypothesis.

Screening protocols for breast and ovarian cancers: Women are advised to examine their own breasts after a period each month, and to seek medical advice if they see or feel any changes.

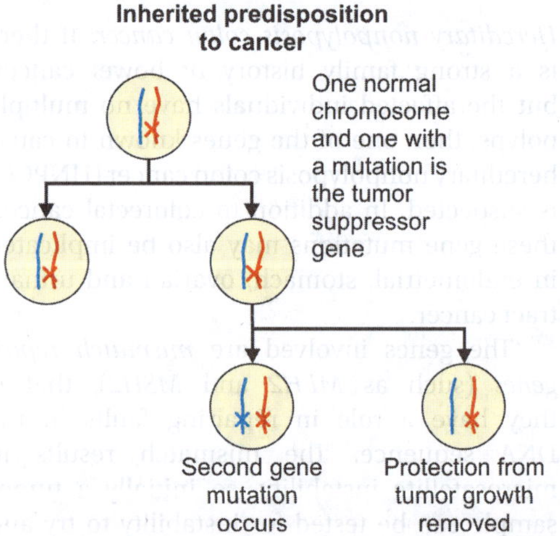

FIGURE 19.1 Two-hit hypothesis

Mammography is used extensively, and at present is the screening method of choice, but is less sensitive in premenopausal women than in those who are postmenopausal, and so is less effective in the high-risk group for whom additional screening is needed.

Similarly, ovarian screening is not highly sensitive. Ultrasound of the ovaries is used, but may not detect a tumor. The CA125 test, which is a measurement of a hormone excreted when there is a malignancy in the ovary, may also be used, and if there is a suspicion of a tumor on ultrasound or CA125 testing, an ovarian biopsy has to be performed.

COLORECTAL CANCER

Familial adenomatous polyposis (FAP)—also called polyposis coli: Owing to a change in the *APC* gene, multiple polyps grow inside the colon. These predispose to adenocarcinoma of the colon or rectum. If a person has the gene mutation, they are almost certain to develop hundreds of polyps in their teens or 20s. Family members who are at risk should be screened annually by colonoscopy, from early adolescence (10–12 years). If a person develops multiple polyps, colectomy is performed to reduce the cancer risk, often in the late teens. Every child of an affected person has a 50 percent chance of inheriting the condition.

Hereditary nonpolyposis colon cancer: If there is a strong family history of bowel cancer, but the affected individuals have no multiple polyps, then one of the genes known to cause hereditary nonpolyposis colon cancer (HNPCC) is suspected. In addition to colorectal cancer, these gene mutations may also be implicated in endometrial, stomach, ovarian and urinary tract cancer.

The genes involved are *mismatch repair genes* (such as *MLH2* and *MSH2*), that is they have a role in repairing faults in the DNA sequence. The mismatch results in microsatellite instability, so initially a tumor sample can be tested for instability to try and locate the site of the gene mutation.

Regular screening by colonoscopy from about 25 years of age is recommended if a person is at risk of HNPCC.

Colorectal cancer predisposition: There are a number of families, where there is some evidence for the presence of a gene mutation, but the cancers in the family may also have occurred sporadically. In these families, screening may be undertaken on a less frequent basis, for example every 5 years.

PRESYMPTOMATIC GENETIC TESTING IN FAMILIAL CANCER

In both familial breast and bowel cancer, there may be a number of potential genes involved, and the mutation may differ from family to family. It is, therefore, necessary to identify the faulty gene in each family before genetic testing can be offered to unaffected family members. Samples from an affected person are required for analysis, and only when the gene mutation is found, presymptomatic testing can be offered to others in the family.

Inborn Errors of Metabolism

The term inborn error of metabolism was coined by a British physician, Archibald Garrod (1857–1936), in the early 20th century (1908). He is known for work that prefigured the "one gene, one enzyme" hypothesis, based on his studies on the nature and inheritance of alkaptonuria.

Inborn errors of metabolism comprise a large class of genetic diseases involving disorders of metabolism. The majority are due to defects of single genes that code for enzymes that facilitate conversion of various substances (substrates) into others (products). In most of the disorders, problems arise due to accumulation of substances which are toxic or interfere with normal function, or to the effects of reduced ability to synthesize essential compounds. Inborn errors of metabolism are now often referred to as congenital metabolic diseases or inherited metabolic diseases.

Major Categories of Inherited Metabolic Diseases

Traditionally, the inherited metabolic diseases were categorized as disorders of carbohydrate metabolism, amino acid metabolism, organic acid metabolism, or lysosomal storage diseases. In recent decades, hundreds of new inherited disorders of metabolism have been discovered and the categories have proliferated. Following are some of the major classes of congenital metabolic diseases, with important examples of each class:

- Disorders of carbohydrate metabolism, e.g. glycogen storage disease
- Disorders of amino acid metabolism, e.g. phenylketonuria, maple syrup urine disease, glutaric acidemia type 1
- Disorders of organic acid metabolism (organic acidurias), e.g. alkaptonuria
- Disorders of fatty acid oxidation and mitochondrial metabolism, e.g. medium chain acyl dehydrogenase deficiency (glutaric acidemia type 2)
- Disorders of porphyrin metabolism, e.g. acute intermittent porphyria
- Disorders of purine or pyrimidine metabolism, e.g. Lesch-Nyhan syndrome
- Disorders of steroid metabolism, e.g. congenital adrenal hyperplasia
- Disorders of mitochondrial function, e.g. Kearns-Sayre syndrome
- Disorders of peroxisomal function, e.g. Zellweger syndrome
- Lysosomal storage disorders, e.g. Gaucher's disease, e.g. Niemann Pick disease.

Manifestations and Presentations

The following are examples of potential manifestations affecting each of the major organ systems:

Growth failure, failure to thrive, weight loss, ambiguous genitalia, delayed puberty, precocious puberty, developmental delay, seizures, dementia, encephalopathy, stroke, deafness, blindness, pain, agnosia, skin rash, abnormal pigmentation, lack of pigmentation, excessive hair growth, dental abnormalities, immunodeficiency, thrombocytopenia, anemia, enlarged spleen, enlarged lymph nodes, many forms of cancer, recurrent vomiting, diarrhea, abdominal pain, excessive urination, renal failure, dehydration, edema, hypotension, heart failure, enlarged heart, hypertension, myocardial infarction, hepatomegaly, jaundice, liver failure, unusual facial features, congenital malformations, excessive breathing (hyperventilation), respiratory failure, abnormal behavior, depression, psychosis, joint pain, muscle weakness, cramps, hypothyroidism, adrenal insufficiency, hypogonadism, diabetes mellitus.

Diagnostic Techniques

Because of the multiplicity of conditions, many different diagnostic tests are used for screening. An abnormal result is often followed by a subsequent "definitive test" to confirm the suspected diagnosis.

Common Screening Tests Used

- Ferric chloride test (turns colors in reaction to various abnormal metabolites in urine)
- Ninhydrin paper chromatography (detects abnormal amino acid patterns)
- Guthrie bacterial inhibition assay (detects a few amino acids in excessive amounts in blood). The dried blood spot can be used for multianalyte testing using Tandem Mass Spectroscopy (MS/MS)
- Quantitative plasma amino acids, quantitative urine amino acids
- Urine organic acids by mass spectrometry.

Blood Group Alleles and Hematological Disorders

The most well-known and medically important blood types are in the ABO group. They were discovered in 1900 and 1901 at the University of Vienna by *Karl Landsteiner* in the process of trying to learn why blood transfusions sometimes cause death and at other times save

a patient. There are four principal types: A, B, AB, and O. There are two antigens and two antibodies that are mostly responsible for the ABO types. The specific combination of these four components determines an individual's type in most cases (Table 19.1).

GENETIC INHERITANCE PATTERNS

The ABO blood types are inherited through genes on chromosome 9, and they do not change as a result of environmental influences during life. An individual's ABO type is determined by the inheritance of 1 of 3 alleles (A, B, or O) from each parent. The possible outcomes are listed in Table 19.2.

Both A and B alleles are dominant over O. As a result, individuals who have an AO genotype will have an A phenotype. People who are type O have OO genotypes. In other words, they inherited a recessive O allele from both parents. The A and B alleles are codominant. Therefore, if an A is inherited from one parent and a B from the other, the phenotype will be AB. Agglutination tests will show that these individuals have the characteristics of both type A and type B blood.

TABLE 19.1 Possible permutations of antigens and antibodies with the corresponding ABO type ("yes" indicates the presence of a component and "no" indicates its absence in the blood of an individual)

ABO blood type	*Antigen A*	*Antigen B*	*Antibody anti-A*	*Antibody anti-B*
A	Yes	No	No	Yes
B	No	Yes	Yes	No
O	No	No	Yes	Yes
AB	Yes	Yes	No	No

TABLE 19.2 The possible ABO alleles for one parent are in the top row and the alleles of the other are in the left column. Offspring genotypes are shown in black. Phenotypes are green

Parent alleles	*A*	*B*	*O*
A	AA(A)	AB(AB)	AO(A)
B	AB(AB)	BB(B)	BO(B)
O	AO	BO	OO

Other Blood Groups

The other blood type of importance is Rh factor. This has only two alleles, one dominant (Rh-positive) and one recessive (Rh-negative). During reproduction, Rh-negative mothers who bear Rh-positive babies may react to them.

GENETIC HEMATOLOGICAL DISORDERS

Sickle-cell Disease

Sickle-cell disease, or sickle-cell anemia (or drepanocytosis), is a life-long blood disorder characterized by red blood cells that assume an abnormal, rigid, sickle shape. Sickling decreases the cells' flexibility and results in a risk of various complications. The sickling occurs because of a mutation in the hemoglobin gene.

Pathophysiology

Sickle-cell anemia is caused by a point mutation in the β-globin chain of hemoglobin, causing the hydrophilic amino acid glutamic acid to be replaced with the hydrophobic amino acid valine at the sixth position. The β-globin gene is found on the short arm of chromosome 11. The association of two wild-type β-globin subunits with two mutant β-globin subunits forms hemoglobin S (HbS). Under low-oxygen conditions (being at high altitude, for example), the absence of a polar amino acid at position six of the β-globin chain promotes the non-covalent polymerization (aggregation) of hemoglobin, which distorts red blood cells into a sickle shape and decreases their elasticity.

The loss of red blood cell elasticity is central to the pathophysiology of sickle-cell disease.

Normal red blood cells are quite elastic, which allows the cells to deform to pass through capillaries. In sickle-cell disease, low-oxygen tension promotes red blood cell sickling and repeated episodes of sickling damage the cell membrane and decreases the cell's elasticity. These cells fail to return to normal shape when normal oxygen tension is restored. As a consequence, these rigid blood cells are unable to deform as they pass through narrow capillaries, leading to vessel occlusion and ischemia.

The actual anemia of the illness is caused by hemolysis, the destruction of the red cells inside the spleen, because of their mis-shape. Although the bone marrow attempts to compensate by creating new red cells, it does not match the rate of destruction. Healthy red blood cells typically live 90 to 120 days, but sickle cells only survive 10 to 20 days.

Genetics

In people heterozygous for HgbS (carriers of sickling hemoglobin), the polymerization problems are minor, because the normal allele is able to produce over 50 percent of the hemoglobin. In people homozygous for HgbS, the presence of long-chain polymers of HbS distort the shape of the red blood cell from a smooth donut-like shape to ragged and full of spikes, making it fragile and susceptible to breaking within capillaries. Carriers have symptoms only if they are deprived of oxygen (for example, while climbing a mountain) or while severely dehydrated. The sickle-cell disease occurs when the glutamic acid, is replaced by valine to change its structure and function.

The gene defect is a known mutation of a single nucleotide of the β-globin gene, which results in glutamate being substituted by valine at position 6. Hemoglobin S with this mutation are referred to as HbS, as opposed to the normal adult HbA. The genetic disorder is due to the mutation of a single nucleotide, from a GAG to GTG codon mutation. This is normally a benign mutation, causing no apparent effects on the secondary, tertiary, or quaternary structure of hemoglobin in conditions of normal oxygen concentration. What it does allow for, under conditions of low-oxygen concentration, is the polymerization of the HbS itself. The deoxy form of hemoglobin exposes a hydrophobic patch on the protein between the E and F helices. The hydrophobic residues of the valine at position 6 of the beta chain in hemoglobin are able to associate with the hydrophobic patch, causing hemoglobin S molecules to aggregate and form fibrous precipitates.

The allele responsible for sickle-cell anemia is autosomal incomplete dominant and can be found on the short arm of chromosome 11. A person that receives the defective gene from both father and mother develops the disease; a person that receives one defective and one healthy allele remains healthy, but can pass on the disease and is known as a carrier. If two parents who are carriers have a child, there is a 1-in-4 chance of their child's developing the disease and a 1-in-2 chance of their child's being just a carrier. Since the gene is incompletely recessive, carriers can produce a few sickled red blood cells, not enough to cause symptoms, but enough to give resistance to malaria. Because of this, heterozygotes have a higher fitness than either of the homozygotes. This is known as heterozygote advantage.

The malaria parasite has a complex life cycle and spends part of it in red blood cells. In a carrier, the presence of the malaria parasite causes the red blood cells with defective hemoglobin to rupture prematurely, making the plasmodium unable to reproduce. Further, the polymerization of Hb affects the ability of the parasite to digest Hb. Therefore, in areas where malaria is a problem, people's chances of survival actually increase if they carry sickle-cell trait (selection for the heterozygote).

Inheritance

Sickle-cell conditions are inherited from parents in much the same way as blood type, hair color and texture, eye color, and other physical traits.

The types of hemoglobin a person makes in the red blood cells depend on what hemoglobin genes are inherited from his parents.

- If one parent has sickle-cell anemia (SS) and the other has sickle-cell trait (AS), there is a 50 percent chance of a child's having sickle-cell disease (SS) and a 50 percent chance of a child's having sickle-cell trait (AS).
- When both parents have sickle-cell trait (AS), a child has a 25 percent chance (1 of 4) of sickle-cell disease (SS), as shown in the diagram (Fig. 19.2).

HEMOPHILIA

Hemophilia is a group of hereditary genetic disorders that impair the body's ability to control blood clotting or coagulation, which is used to stop bleeding when a blood vessel is broken. Hemophilia A is a recessive X-linked genetic disorder involving a lack of functional clotting factor VIII and represents 90 percent of hemophilia cases, occurring at about 1 in 5,000 to 10,000 male births. Hemophilia B is a recessive X-linked genetic disorder involving a lack of functional clotting factor IX. It is similar to but less common than hemophilia A. Hemophilia C is an autosomal genetic disorder (i.e. not X-linked) involving a lack of functional clotting factor XI. Hemophilia C is not completely recessive. Heterozygous individuals also show increased bleeding.

Similar to most recessive sex-linked, X chromosome disorders, only males typically exhibit symptoms. This is due to the fact that females have two X chromosomes while males have only one, lacking a 'backup' copy for the defective gene the defective gene becomes manifest more easily in males. Because females have two X chromosomes and because hemophilia is rare, the chance of a female having two defective copies of the gene is

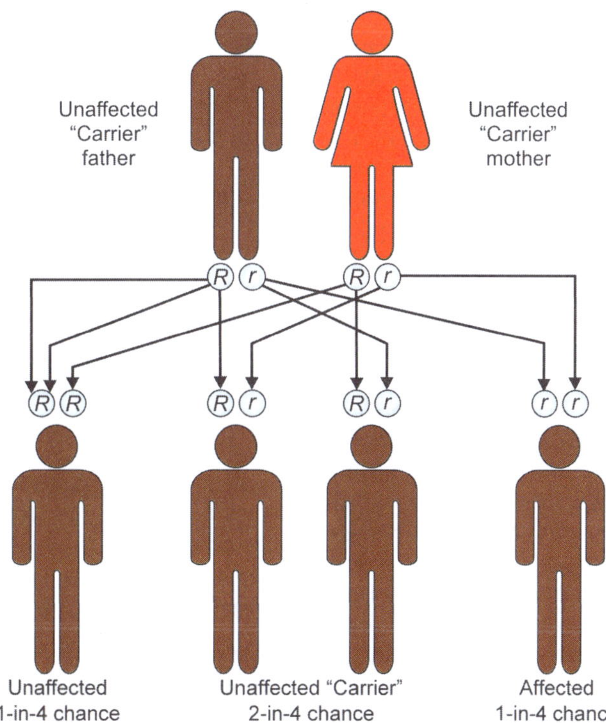

FIGURE 19.2 Sickle-cell disease is inherited in the autosomal recessive pattern

very low, thus females are almost exclusively asymptomatic carriers of the disorder. Female carriers may inherit the defective gene from either their mother, father, or it may be a new mutation. Only under rare circumstances do females actually have hemophilia. Affected males typically inherit the defective gene from their mother, or it can be a new mutation.

Hemophiliacs do not bleed more intensely than a normal person, but can bleed for a much longer amount of time. In severe hemophiliacs even a minor injury could result in blood loss lasting days, weeks, or not ever healing completely. In areas such as the brain or inside joints, this can be fatal or permanently debilitating.

Genetics

Females possess two X chromosomes, males have one X and one Y chromosome. Since the mutations causing the disease are recessive, a woman carrying the defect on one of her X chromosomes may not be affected by it, as the equivalent allele on her other chromosome should express itself to produce the necessary clotting factors. However, the Y chromosome in men has no gene for factors VIII or IX. If the genes responsible for production of factor VIII or factor IX present on a male's X chromosome are deficient there is no equivalent on the Y chromosome, so the deficient gene is not masked by the dominant allele and he will develop the illness.

Since a male receives his single X chromosome from his mother, the son of a healthy female silently carrying the deficient gene will have a 50 percent chance of inheriting that gene from her and with it the disease; and if his mother is affected with hemophilia, he will have a 100 percent chance of being a hemophiliac. In contrast, for a female to inherit the disease, she must receive two deficient X chromosomes, one from her mother and the other from her father (who must, therefore, be a hemophiliac himself). Hence hemophilia is far more common among males than females. However, it is possible for female carriers to become mild hemophiliacs due to lyonization (inactivation) of the X chromosomes. Hemophiliac daughters are more common than they once were, as improved treatments for the disease have allowed more hemophiliac males to survive to adulthood and become parents. Adult females may experience menorrhagia (heavy periods) due to the bleeding tendency. The pattern of inheritance is criss-cross type. This type of pattern is also seen in color blindness.

A mother who is a carrier has a 50 percent chance of passing the faulty X chromosome to her daughter, while an affected father will always pass on the affected gene to his daughters. A son cannot inherit the defective gene from his father (Fig. 19.3).

Genetic testing and genetic counseling is recommended for families with hemophilia. Prenatal testing, such as amniocentesis, is available to pregnant women who may be carriers of the condition. As with all genetic disorders, it is also possible for a human to acquire it spontaneously through mutation, rather than inheriting it, because of a new mutation in one of their parents' gametes. Spontaneous mutations account for about 33 percent of all cases of hemophilia A. About 30 percent of cases of hemophilia B are the result of a spontaneous gene mutation.

GENETIC HEMOCHROMATOSIS

Genetic hemochromatosis is an autosomal recessive inherited disorder of iron metabolism. It is a treatable adult-onset disorder and screening is possible either using measures of serum iron, transferrin saturation or using a genetic test.

The gene *(HFE)* was identified in 1996 and two common mutations are shown to account for 90 percent of cases. Most affected people have two copies of a mutation called C282Y; a small proportion have the C282Y mutation together with a mutation called H63D. The genetic predisposition leads to accumulation of body iron stores over time.

Complications include cirrhosis, primary liver cancer, cardiomyopathy, arthritis and

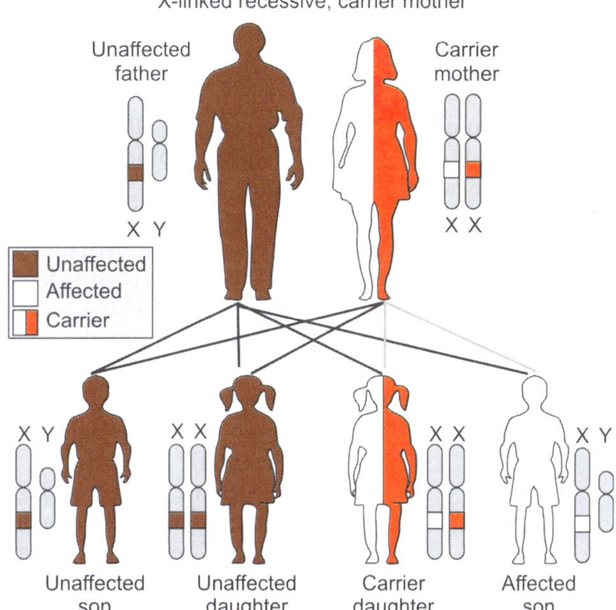

FIGURE 19.3 Inheritance of hemophilia

diabetes when iron overload is sufficient to cause organ damage. Treatment for the condition involves removing multiple units of blood until the body iron stores return to normal. A maintenance program of venesection is then needed to prevent reaccumulation of iron. This treatment prolongs survival in symptomatic people and appears to restore normal life expectancy if started early enough in the course of the disease.

Specific diagnostic tests (or focused screening for a small set of disorders):

- Tissue biopsy or necropsy: Liver, muscle, brain, bone marrow
- Skin biopsy and fibroblast cultivation for specific enzyme testing
- Specific DNA testing.

Huntington's Disease

George Huntington first described the condition in the literature in 1872 that the disease is dominantly inherited, the mutation was identified in 1993.

'Anticipation' refers to the phenomenon in which succeeding generations of the family develop the disease at a younger age than the preceding generation. In families affected by HD, anticipation sometimes occurs. The mutation in the *huntingtin* gene is an expansion, that is, abnormal genes are longer than the normal gene. In the genetic material, certain base pair sequences are often repeated within a gene. Within the *huntingtin* gene, unaffected individuals have up to 35 repeated copies of the sequence 'CAG'. However, affected patients have more than 35 copies of the CAG triplet in one allele of the gene. They, thus, have one normal and one expanded copy of the gene.

The CAG trinucleotide codes for glutamine, and the expanded gene increases the length of a glutamine chain in the cell cytoplasm, causing it to form clumps and invade the nucleus of the cell. This results in premature death of brain cells. Once the number of CAG repeats in the gene has expanded, it is less stable and the number of repeats can increase when the gene is copied during meiosis. The expansion is

more likely to increase during spermatogenesis than oogenesis. Hence, if a man has HD, his children may inherit a larger copy of the gene than he has, and develop the condition at an earlier age.

The signs and symptoms of HD vary with each individual, but fall into three main groups:

- *Physical disability:* The first physical signs may be clumsiness, stumbling and unsteadiness. Eventually, chorea may be evident, and walking becomes very difficult. The speech becomes slurred.
- *Mental disability:* Initially, the patient is often aware that their memory is becoming worse, especially short-term memory. Some patients eventually suffer serious dementia.
- *Psychiatric problems:* Depression may be the first sign of HD, and can be treated with antidepressants. Paranoia and obsessive behavior may also be present.

MENTAL ILLNESS

Affective Disorder (Manic Depression)

This is a term used to cover manic depression or depression alone. Studies indicate that the earlier the age at which a person is affected, the more likely it is that relatives will also be affected. However, the only basis upon which to advise a patient inquiring about their own risk is the data collected on families. These data enable a risk figure to be given, ranging from a risk of 5 percent if a second-degree relative has manic depression, to a risk of about 50 percent if both parents of the patient have been affected.

Schizophrenia

From some studies, it is clear that there is an increased risk of schizophrenia to relatives of an affected person. The genetic link is demonstrated, when we consider the incidence of schizophrenia in twins. When one twin is affected, 40 percent of monozygotic twin siblings are also affected, as compared with only 10 percent of dizygotic twin siblings. This indicates that even after allowing for a common environment, the concordance between those who inherit identical genetic material risk is high.

Again, the risk is high (45%) if both parents of the patient are schizophrenic.

It is important when advising families of their risk to try to confirm the diagnosis in the affected person. Some inherited neurological conditions, such as Huntington's disease may present with a severe psychiatric illness, but of course the risk to the patient may be very different.

Presenile Dementia (Early Alzheimer's Disease)

Presenile dementia is a condition (like breast or bowel cancer) that may occur sporadically, or may be caused by a gene mutation. Generally, late-onset Alzheimer's disease will be due to old age, rather than an inherited mutation, but if there is a history of dementia occurring in several younger members of a family, this may be connected with a mutation in one of the *presenilin* genes. Where a gene mutation exists, children of an affected parent will be at 50 percent risk of inheriting the mutation and developing early dementia.

CHAPTER 20

Service Related to Genetics

GENETIC TESTING

Genetic testing is done on such material as blood, hair, skin, amniotic fluid or any other tissue. The DNA in the samples is analyzed for a particular disorder. Screening of the newborn baby is done for congenital anomalies using blood sample, taken by pricking baby's heel.

Before any genetic testing is done, the concerned person is informed and made to understand the procedure of the tests, limitations of the test and the possible consequences of the test result. This process of educating an individual about the test and taking permission is called *Informed consent.*

HUMAN GENOME PROJECT

A genome is the complete set of DNA of an organism. Each genome contains all the information needed to build and maintain that organism.

The human genome project was a large scale international research effort to determine the sequence of the human genome and identify the genes that it contains. The project was coordinated by the National Institutes of Health and the U.S. Department of Energy. The project began in 1990 and was completed in 2003. Each and every gene in the human genome was unraveled to its perfection. This project gave us an important blueprint for building a person.

Goals of Human Genome Project

The important goals of human genome project were:

- To provide a complete and accurate sequence of all the DNA in the human genome
- To find all the estimated 20,000 to 25,000 human genes.

The project also aimed at sequencing the genomes of other organisms important in medical research, such as mouse and the fruit fly.

Accomplishments of Human Genome Project

It was in April 2003, that the mapping of entire human genome was complete. It bridged the gap in the working draft of the genome, which was published in 2001. Also identified were the genomes of fruit fly, roundworm and Brewer's yeast. The project's ethical, legal and social implications (ELSI) program became the world's largest bioethics program and a model for other ELSI program worldwide.

Ethical, Legal and Social Implications of Human Genome Project

The ELSI program was an integral part of human genome project. The aims of the ELSI program

were to identify and address issues raised by genomic research that would affect individuals, families and society.

The ELSI program focused on the possible consequences of genomic research in four main areas:

- Privacy and fairness in the use of genetic information, including the potential for genetic discrimination in employment and insurance.
- The integration of new genetic technologies, such as genetic testing, into the practice of clinical medicine.
- Ethical issues surrounding the design and conduct of genetic research with people, including the process of informed consent.
- The education of health care professionals, policy makers, students and the public about genetics and complex issues that result from genomic research.

Future Perspectives of Genomic Research

Discovering the sequence of the human genome was only the stepping stone of genetics. The research later includes deducing the different mutations and the novel approach to treat them with gene therapy.

The objectives of continued genomic research include:

- Determine the function of genes and the elements that regulate genes throughout the genome.
- Find variations in the DNA sequence among people and determine their significance.
- Discover the three-dimensional structures of proteins and identify their functions.
- Explore the interaction of DNA and proteins.
- Develop and apply genome based strategies for the early detection, diagnosis and treatment of disease.
- Sequence the genomes of other organisms.
- Develop new technologies to study genes and DNA on a large-scale and store genomic data efficiently.
- Continue to explore the ethical, legal and social issues raised by genomic research.

GENE THERAPY

Gene therapy is the therapeutic application of the knowledge of genetics. Many hereditary diseases due to mutant allele can be treated with the replacement of the mutant allele by a functional one.

The basic process of gene therapy involved the insertion of a normal functional gene to replace the abnormal mutant gene. This requires a carrier vector to deliver the therapeutic gene to the patient's target cells. The most commonly used vectors are viruses which have been produced by genetic engineering to carry the functional gene.

Types of Gene Therapy

- *Germ line gene therapy:* In this, the sperms or the ova are modified by the introduction of functional genes, which are ordinarily integrated into their genomes. So, now the change due to modification would be heritable and would be passed on to later generation. This novel approach would help to combat a number of inherited genetic diseases. But, due to technical and ethical constraints, this type of gene therapy is not used in humans.
- *Somatic cell gene therapy*: This involves the introduction of functional gene into the somatic cells, especially in those tissues in which expression of the concerned gene is critical for health. Expression of the introduced gene relieves the symptoms in that particular individual, but it is not heritable, as the germ cells are not involved. In the present scenario, somatic gene therapy is a good option and clinical and field trials have already begun in this line.

Vectors in Gene Therapy

Viruses: One of the steps in the replication cycle of the viruses is the integration of their genetic

material within the host genome. This will alter the host genome to produce more and more copies of the virus.

This property of genetic integration on the viral genetic material into the host cell genome is exploited in gene therapy. The viruses are used to carry functional genes as vectors into the human cell. This results in the integration of the functional genes of the vector with the human cell genome to get the desired effect.

Retroviruses, adenoviruses and adeno-associated viruses have been used as vectors for gene therapy.

Nonviral Methods

The nonviral methods have the advantage of large-scale production.

- *Naked DNA:* The naked DNA plasmids have been used but with limited success.
- *Oligonucleotides:* Specific oligonucleotides are synthesized that act to inactivate the genes involved in a disease process.
- *Lipoplexes and polyplexes:* Lipoplexes and apoplexes confer protection to the DNA to protect it against degradation during transfection.

The Eugenics Movement

The Eugenics Society was born of Galton's ideas. A Bill concerning voluntary sterilization for those in the Social Problem Group was drafted by the Brock Committee in 1934, but did not become legislation. One of the aims of the Eugenics Society was to make affordable contraceptive methods available to those who wished to have them, but the Brock Committee legislation differed in that it was based on a judgment of fitness rather than personal choice. In 1933, a compulsory sterilization law was passed, which included those with hereditary deafness, blindness and Huntington's disease among other congenital disabilities. Later in the same decade, these disabilities became grounds for extermination under the same regime.

Genetic Counseling Legal and Ethical Issues—Role of Nurse

The four main components of the role of genetic counselor are:

1. Communication with patients, both to obtain the family medical history necessary to provide the patient with reliable information, convey the genetic information, and present the options available to the family in a nonjudgmental manner.
2. Patient support, particularly at times of decision-making or particular stress, e.g. after a new diagnosis has been made in the family, during an at-risk pregnancy or when testing is being considered.
3. Education of patients and other health professionals on issues related to clinical genetics.
4. Skilled interpretation of current research findings for the benefit of patients.

Ethical Practice

The genetic counselor is able to:

- Recognize and maintain professional boundaries
- Demonstrate reflective skills within the counseling context and in personal awareness for the safety of patients and families by participation in counseling/clinical supervision
- Practice in accordance with the AGNC Code of Ethical Conduct
- Present opportunities for clients to participate in research projects in a manner that facilitates informed choice
- Recognize his or her own limitations in knowledge and capabilities and discuss with colleagues or refer patients when necessary
- Demonstrate continuing professional development as an individual practitioner and for the development of the profession
- Contribute to the development and organization of genetic services.

The Association of Genetic Nurses and Counselors in the UK has established a formal

registration process for genetic counselors. A code of ethics has been adopted, and the registration system is based upon a set of competency standards, which are the knowledge, skills and attitudes necessary to enable a practitioner to function effectively and safely in a specific field of activity. Standards of competence facilitate the regulation of practitioners and provide a useful basis for devising educational pathways that are directly applicable to the skills required for the work.

It is apparent that the demand for genetic services will increase as technology offers more in the form of genetic testing, pharmacogenetics and possibly gene therapy. In addition to the rare genetic disorders, genetic services may also be required to make a contribution to the health care of those with common conditions in which there is a genetic component. This may not be direct care for patients with those conditions, but will almost certainly involve providing education and consultation for other health care professionals.

The genetic counselor needs to be educated sufficiently to interpret the complex scientific data for the benefit of patients, and to possess the counseling skills to ensure patients can express their opinions, explore the options and make informed decisions.

As consumers become more aware of the availability of genetic counseling and testing, genetic counselors must be prepared to provide a certain standard of service.

Index

Page nimbers followed by *f* refer to figure and *t* refer to table

D

E

F

G

H

I

J

K

L

R

S

T

Textbook of

PATHOLOGY AND GENETICS

for BSc Nursing Students